Healing Toxic Relationships

Six Secrets to Building Healthy Relationships After a Toxic Family

Steven Todd Bryant

I0704955

Disclaimer

This book is not intended as a substitute for the medical advice of physicians. The reader must consult a physician in matters relating to his/her/their health and particularly with respect to any symptoms that may require diagnosis or medical attention. Although the author has made every effort to ensure the information in this book was correct at press time, the author does not assume and hereby disclaims any liability to any party for any loss, damage, or disruption caused by errors or omissions for any reason. The author cannot be held legally responsible for any damages suffered because of this publication or the content of 3rd party web pages or resources. In some cases, stories have been fictionalized, and names and identifying details have been omitted or changed to protect the privacy of individuals.

Table of Contents

About the Author

Steven Todd Bryant is a best-selling author, crisis counselor, toxic family survivor, and founder of ToxicFamily.org. An expert in toxic family dynamics, he spent 19 years on staff at the University of Southern California and holds an MA in Theological Studies. He resides in Southern California.

Follow Steven Todd Bryant
facebook.com/StevenToddBryant
amazon.com/author/steventoddbryant
www.steventoddbryant.com/

Books by Steven Todd Bryant
Healing Toxic Relationships
The Toxic Family Solution
Unclutter Your Life to Find Meaning & Purpose
The Wisdom of Swedish Death Cleaning
Healing Toxic Love
Toxic Family 365

Dedication

Dedicated to all those struggling to overcome a toxic family—may you find hope in knowing that your future is brighter than your past.

In a toxic relationship, it often feels like no matter what you do, you're always in the wrong. Just when you think you've figured out how to navigate the toxic family dynamics, the rules change, leaving you feeling unsettled and off-balance. Toxic relationships create a relentless cycle of confusion, where validation, security, and intimacy are constantly out of reach. Sometimes, in a toxic family, the only way to win is not to play.

Breaking free from toxic family dynamics starts with discovering the secrets to healing. One of these secrets is letting go of the behaviors that once helped you cope but now harm your adult relationships. Sometimes, it also means distancing yourself from people who continue to cause pain, creating space for your own healing and growth. The ways you learned to navigate dysfunction as a child—whether by keeping the peace, hiding your true feelings or always being on guard—were essential for survival. However, as an adult, these behaviors can prevent you from living your best life.

The secrets I learned from surviving my own toxic family will help you reclaim your sense of self, break free from the destructive patterns of your past, and start building healthier, more fulfilling intimate relationships today. These insights will empower you to move beyond the defense mechanisms that once protected you but now hold you back, set strong boundaries that foster emotional safety, and cultivate meaningful connections rooted in mutual respect and trust. You are about to discover how to release fear and insecurity and finally live the life of connection, happiness, and joy you truly deserve.

By acknowledging and addressing the toxic influences from your family, you can begin to unravel the harmful patterns of manipulation, control, and emotional turmoil they imposed on you. This journey involves not only understanding how these behaviors were shaped by your upbringing but also developing new, healthier ways of coping and relating to others. As you move forward, you'll discover greater emotional freedom, stability, and the ability to build more authentic, fulfilling relationships—ones grounded in mutual respect, trust, and intimacy rather than fear or control.

Walking away from dysfunctional behavior or harmful individuals is never easy, but when intimate relationships cause pain, stress, self-doubt, and insecurity, it's essential to reassess their impact on your well-being. You deserve a life filled with fulfilling relationships, peace, and joy. It's time for you to reevaluate your unhealthy relationships and start living your best life now.

Healing Toxic Relationships: Six Secrets to Building Healthy Relationships After a Toxic Family explores how growing up in a toxic family can deeply affect your adult relationships. Early dysfunctional experiences often shape how you approach intimacy and connection, leading you to unconsciously seek out toxic dynamics while struggling with boundaries and maintaining your sense of self. This timely book offers principles to help you recognize these patterns, break free from harmful cycles, and build healthier, more fulfilling connections. You deserve relationships that uplift and empower you—not drag you down—and it's entirely possible to heal from the past and find relationships that strengthen, rather than diminish, who you truly are.

Healing Toxic Relationships is for anyone ready to escape the toxic cycles inherited from an unhealthy family and begin the journey toward emotional freedom and authentic relationships. Whether you're healing old wounds, strengthening an existing relationship, or creating new, healthier connections, this book provides the tools for meaningful transformations in your closest relationships, empowering you to live your best life, full of fulfillment, joy, and peace.

My Story

My father always said he loved me, but his actions painted a much darker picture. For eighteen years, I lived in a home saturated with domestic violence, where verbal, emotional, psychological, and spiritual abuse were relentless, tearing through every moment of my daily life. Each day, I braced myself for his rage, terrified that his violent words would eventually turn into physical violence.

While I felt loved by my mother, she always sided with my father. She excused, enabled, and defended his destructive behavior, leaving me feeling betrayed and isolated. The hopes I had for a happy family and a nurturing childhood were never realized. Even after leaving my toxic family, I realized the damaging wounds of those early relationships ran deep.

Growing up in this environment robbed me of the sense of safety and connection every child deserves. Instead of feeling secure, I learned to walk on eggshells, constantly bracing for the next outburst. My brain shifted into survival mode, becoming hypervigilant, always scanning for signs of danger. I developed coping mechanisms that helped me get through the day but left deep emotional scars. Over time, I began to confuse connection with fear, internalizing the belief that relationships are built on power, control, and terror.

My constant state of fear and anxiety not only robbed me of my childhood but also shattered my sense of self-worth. It eroded my ability to trust others and left me questioning the reliability and security of close relationships. These deep emotional wounds followed me into adulthood, profoundly shaping how I navigated my most intimate connections.

After years of failed adult relationships, my journey of healing truly began to flourish after four years of psychotherapy, self-reflection, and developing practical strategies to overcome the negative patterns ingrained by my family. Additionally, I learned how to meditate and practice mindfulness, which helped me to regulate my emotions and stay present in the moment. This transformation has given me profound empathy and insight into the struggles of others.

I was trained as a crisis counselor and began helping individuals struggling with suicidal thoughts, many of whom were grappling with the trauma caused by toxic family environments. During this time, I founded ToxicFamily.org to provide resources and support for individuals dealing with the aftermath of toxic family dynamics. This website has reached countless people, offering hope and practical tools for healing.

In therapy, I confronted the deep, long-standing wounds of my past and began the challenging and transformative process of unlearning the toxic patterns I inherited from my family. This journey wasn't quick or easy, but it allowed me to gain a profound understanding of my emotional landscape and how my upbringing shaped my adult relationships. Therapy helped me realize that many of my struggles with identity, self-worth, trust, and intimacy were rooted in the dynamics of my abusive childhood. Additionally, the years I spent numbing myself with addictive substances began to lose their grip as I came to terms with my toxic past.

What began as a personal journey to healing my own wounds has evolved into a lifelong mission to support others on similar paths. This book is the culmination of the key principles I've learned about strengthening intimate relationships after healing the deep scars left by a toxic family. *Healing Toxic Relationships* explores topics rarely addressed in other toxic family books, uncovering the deep secrets to overcoming toxic family dynamics and transforming lives affected by the painful emotional scars that unhealthy family environments leave behind.

What to Expect from *Healing Toxic Relationships*
Healing Toxic Relationships provides a practical roadmap for recovering from the emotional wounds of a toxic family by transforming how you view your past, yourself, your intimate relationships, and your connections. Each chapter addresses important challenges and provides specific ways to shift your mindset for healing and growth.

Here is a preview of the topics we'll be discussing. This book's content is designed to help you shift the unhealthy perspectives shaped by your toxic family, break free from limiting thought patterns, and cultivate healthier, more fulfilling relationships.

The Deep Scars of Toxic Family Relationships
Growing up in a toxic family leaves deep emotional scars that shape your self-worth and relationships. Manipulation, neglect, and emotional abuse from childhood continue to impact how you trust others and connect emotionally. We'll explore the long-lasting effects of these experiences and understand how they show up in our adult relationships. This insight provides the foundation to recognize the barriers preventing you from experiencing healthy, meaningful connections and offers the first steps toward healing.

Transcending Automatic Defense Mechanisms in Relationships
In a toxic family environment, many people develop automatic defense mechanisms such as fight, flight, freeze, or fawn to protect themselves from emotional harm. You are likely already familiar with the responses of fight, flight, and freeze. The automatic defense mechanism fawn is the tendency to excessively people-please or appease others to avoid conflict or gain approval, often at the expense of your own needs and boundaries.

While these defense mechanisms may have been helpful in childhood, they can become obstacles to emotional connection in adult relationships. Together, we'll work to recognize these patterns and find ways to overcome them, learning how to engage with your partner* from a place of emotional clarity and resilience, rather than from fear or reactivity.

Throughout this book, the term "partner" is used broadly to refer to any significant relationship in your life—whether it's with a romantic partner, family member, close friend, co-worker, or other important connection.

Embracing Ego Death in Relationships

Growing up in a toxic family often forces us to develop protective mechanisms to shield ourselves from emotional pain. One of these defenses is the ego—the part of us that seeks to protect our self-image by maintaining control, avoiding vulnerability, and keeping others at arm's length. In a toxic family, the unpredictability of emotions and relationships can drive us to focus on being right, winning arguments, or controlling situations in order to feel safe.

Ego death refers to the process of letting go of this need for control and self-preservation in order to experience deeper emotional intimacy. When we release the ego's grip, we allow ourselves to become more open, vulnerable, and authentic in our relationships, no longer ruled by the fear that toxic environments taught us to hold onto.

Letting go of the ego doesn't mean losing who you are. It's about shedding the layers of defensiveness and pride that once served as protection but now prevent true emotional connection. By stepping back from the need to protect or prove yourself constantly, you'll create space for more honest and open communication with your partner. This shift helps build trust and closeness, as both partners feel more seen and understood.

When we focus less on ego-driven behavior and more on sincere, heartfelt connection, our relationships transform. By letting go of control and embracing vulnerability, we can cultivate relationships based on mutual respect, emotional intimacy, and a deeper connection. This approach fosters not only personal growth but also a more fulfilling, authentic partnership.

The Need for Personal Space in Intimate Relationships

In toxic family environments, boundaries are often blurred or ignored entirely, making it difficult to learn the value of personal space. Many people who grew up in these environments mistakenly equate closeness with constant togetherness, believing that distance means detachment or rejection. Without time for personal reflection and emotional recharge, relationships can become suffocating and unbalanced.

We'll explore how growing up in a toxic family can make it hard to establish healthy boundaries and recognize the importance of personal space in adult relationships. By reclaiming your emotional space, you not only honor your individuality but also create a healthier balance between intimacy and independence. This shift strengthens your bond, allowing for deeper, more fulfilling connections with your partner while avoiding the unhealthy enmeshment that toxic family dynamics often create.

Understanding Dependency and Codependency

Toxic family dynamics often breed patterns of dependency or codependency in adult relationships. These imbalances can manifest when one partner becomes overly reliant on the other for emotional security or self-worth. We'll identify the roots of these dynamics and explore how they can hinder emotional independence. Understanding these patterns is crucial to breaking free from unhealthy dependencies and fostering healthier, more equal partnerships. You'll learn how to cultivate a sense of emotional autonomy while still nurturing strong, supportive connections with those you care about.

The ultimate goal of *Healing Toxic Relationships* is to teach you how to form deep connections without losing yourself in the process. Many who come from toxic family environments have learned to equate connection with self-sacrifice, often suppressing their authentic self to keep peace or maintain relationships. This book will help you break that pattern. By applying the principles outlined here, you'll learn how to create relationships that are fulfilling, balanced, and emotionally healthy. The key is understanding that true connection doesn't require sacrificing your true self—it requires self-awareness, strong boundaries, and mutual respect.

The Promise of *Healing Toxic Relationships*

I promise that if you read *Healing Toxic Relationships* from start to finish and diligently apply the insights offered here, you will break free from the harmful patterns instilled by your toxic family background. You'll gain a deeper understanding of the emotional scars left by toxic family dynamics and how they continue to affect your adult relationships. You'll learn to recognize and transcend automatic defense mechanisms that sabotage emotional connection, fostering resilience instead of fear and reactivity.

By embracing the concept of ego death, you'll let go of the need for control and self-preservation, opening yourself up to greater emotional intimacy and authenticity in your relationships. You'll also learn the importance of personal space and independence, understanding how they strengthen, rather than weaken, your bond with others. Finally, you'll confront the challenges of dependency and codependency, cultivating healthier, more balanced connections rooted in mutual respect and emotional freedom.

Start Your Healing Journey Today

There's no need to wait. The journey to healing and building healthy relationships starts right now. You have the power to transform your life and break free from the toxic patterns that have held you back. Every step you take toward understanding and addressing the impact of your past brings you closer to the fulfilling, loving relationships you deserve.

Healing Toxic Relationships is not just a book; it's your guide to a brighter future. The principles and strategies within these pages are carefully designed to empower you with the knowledge and tools you need to make lasting changes. As you read and apply what you learn, you will witness the positive impact on your emotional well-being and your relationships.

Take the first step today. Embrace the opportunity to heal, grow, and discover the connection, joy, and intimacy you've been longing for. The path to building powerful connections and fulfilling relationships is now within your reach. You don't have to walk this journey alone—I'm here to support you every step of the way.

Let's begin this incredible adventure together. Your new life, filled with deep connections, meaningful relationships, and the happiness you deserve, starts now.

—*Steven Todd Bryant*

1. The Deep Scars of Toxic Family Relationships

My father's inconsistent caregiving left deep emotional scars, much of which stemmed from his inability to keep promises. He would often make plans for family gatherings—birthdays, holidays—only to cancel them at the last minute due to anger or drinking too much. His unreliability created a constant sense of uncertainty that made it impossible for me to trust him. This inability to trust and emotional instability lingered throughout my childhood and carried over into my adult relationships.

My toxic family's unpredictability extended even to simple outings, like going to the movies. Every time we went, the event became an ordeal. I remember watching the film while constantly checking to see if my father was enjoying it. Most of the time, before the movie even reached the halfway point, he would loudly declare, "This movie is terrible. We're leaving." Without considering anyone else, he'd storm out, demand refunds for his half-eaten popcorn, and cause a scene at the ticket counter.

Even going out for a meal wasn't safe from my father's unpredictable behavior. Dining with him almost always led to a scene. If the waitstaff looked at him the wrong way, or if the silverware was misplaced, or if the food didn't meet his unreasonable standards, he would explode. I would hold my breath, waiting for him to declare, "We're leaving," and walk out without paying. His outbursts at the staff, combined with his intolerance for even minor inconveniences, turned what should have been a pleasant dinner into an embarrassing, stressful ordeal. Every family outing felt like a potential disaster.

As a child, the constant unpredictability of my father's behavior had a profound psychological impact on me. I developed intense anxiety, always on edge, trying to anticipate his next outburst. The fear of conflict became deeply ingrained, making me hesitant to express my own needs or stand up for myself, afraid that doing so would provoke another episode. Over time, I internalized the message that my feelings were insignificant compared to maintaining peace around him. This created a deep sense of insecurity, leaving me feeling powerless and constantly bracing for the next disaster.

This insecurity followed me into adulthood, where I clung to the false belief that I could control my environment to avoid emotional pain. I eventually realized that while I could manage my own actions and responses, I had little influence over others' behavior or the external circumstances that triggered my anxiety. My futile attempts to manage the uncontrollable only deepened my helplessness when things inevitably went wrong. In my adult relationships, this deep-rooted insecurity manifested as people-pleasing—constantly trying to maintain a fragile peace, always fearing that any calm moment could be shattered.

This trauma shaped how I interacted with others. I became hypervigilant, constantly scanning for signs of displeasure, anger, or rejection. My toxic family taught me that connection and trust were fragile and always at risk of disappearing. The instability I experienced in childhood led to long-lasting mental health challenges, including anxiety and a deep-rooted fear of trusting others. The emotional chaos of my upbringing forced me to walk on eggshells, never knowing where I stood and perpetually uncertain of what to expect in even my closest relationships.

Beyond the emotional and psychological damage, living in

this environment also profoundly impacted my authentic self. Suppressing my needs to avoid conflict gradually caused me to lose touch with who I truly was. Over time, I became disconnected from my identity, with my self-worth tied to how well I could manage others' emotions—an exhausting and impossible task.

This disconnection made it difficult for me to understand what I genuinely wanted from relationships and life, leading to a pattern of self-sacrifice, enabling, and caregiving. Reclaiming my authentic self through mindfulness and therapy has been an ongoing process of unlearning these toxic patterns and rediscovering my voice, free from the fear that shaped so much of my childhood. After enduring 18 years of abuse in my toxic family, it has taken years of psychotherapy and self-reflection to finally feel comfortable in my own skin.

The Long-Term Effects of a Toxic Family

Growing up in a toxic family environment leaves enduring scars that can profoundly affect your emotional well-being and how you relate to others. The behaviors, attitudes, and emotional patterns you develop in such an environment can persist into adulthood, influencing your ability to trust, regulate emotions, and form healthy connections. Becoming aware of these effects is the first step in healing and breaking free from the harmful dynamics that may have shaped your life.

Lack of Trust
Trust is the cornerstone of any healthy relationship, and it extends beyond simply believing in your partner's honesty or dependability. Trust involves feeling safe enough to be vulnerable, knowing that your partner will honor, respect, and support you through life's challenges. It is this trust that creates the emotional security needed for intimacy and lasting connection.

In a toxic family, trust is often shattered early on. Experiences of manipulation, inconsistency, broken promises, or emotional betrayal teach you that people are unreliable. As a child, you may have learned that those who were supposed to care for you were unpredictable or hurtful, which distorts your ability to trust others later in life. This deeply ingrained lack of trust can follow you into adulthood, manifesting as constant suspicion or fear of betrayal in your intimate relationships.

As an adult, you may find yourself doubting your partner's motives or feeling anxious about being hurt, even when there is no real threat. This can lead to possessiveness, jealousy, or even controlling behaviors, all of which undermine the foundation of a relationship. Without trust, it's nearly impossible to build the vulnerability required for genuine intimacy, and this emotional distance can leave you feeling isolated and disconnected, even in close relationships.

Emotional Instability
Emotional stability is the ability to navigate stress and adversity with calm and resilience. It involves managing your emotions in a way that allows you to respond to challenges without being overwhelmed. However, growing up in a toxic family environment often disrupts this ability, leading to emotional instability that can persist into adulthood.

In a toxic family, emotional expressions may have been erratic, intense, or unpredictable. You might have witnessed frequent emotional outbursts, silent treatment, or passive-aggressive behavior. These patterns teach you that emotions are either dangerous or uncontrollable, leading to an internal struggle in managing your own feelings. This emotional turbulence can make it hard to know when or how to express what you're feeling, leaving you either suppressing your emotions or reacting with overwhelming intensity.

As an adult, emotional instability can manifest as frequent mood swings, emotional outbursts, or feelings of emotional numbness.

These ups and downs can create chaos in your relationships, making it difficult to communicate effectively or resolve conflicts. The unpredictability of your emotional responses can leave both you and your partner confused and distressed, eroding the trust and stability that healthy relationships require.

In some cases, emotional instability may also lead to emotional unavailability, a pattern where you withdraw emotionally or avoid deeper connections altogether. If your caregivers didn't model healthy emotional regulation, you may find it challenging to connect emotionally with your partner, creating further distance and dissatisfaction in your relationship.

Perfectionism and Fear of Failure

Another long-term effect of toxic family dynamics is the development of perfectionism and an intense fear of failure. In a toxic family, you might have been expected to meet unrealistic standards or be perfect in order to receive affection and acceptance. This pressure to be flawless can lead to perfectionistic tendencies, where you constantly strive for unattainable goals and become overly critical of yourself when you inevitably fall short.

Perfectionism often presents a false version of who you truly are, as it masks your vulnerabilities and authentic self. By constantly trying to live up to an idealized version of yourself, you not only disconnect from your real emotions and needs, but you also confuse those around you. Others are left responding to the façade of perfection you present, not knowing who you really are or what you genuinely need. This false front prevents you from forming deep, meaningful connections because it becomes impossible for others to meet your emotional needs when they are unaware of your true self.

The impact of perfectionism extends beyond your internal world and into your relationships. You might project these unrealistic standards onto your partner, expecting them to meet the same impossible ideals. This creates tension and resentment, as no one can live up to such high expectations. The fear of failure that accompanies perfectionism can also prevent you from taking risks or being vulnerable in the relationship, stifling emotional growth and spontaneity. Ultimately, perfectionism acts as a barrier, keeping you from fully engaging in and enjoying your relationships while also depriving your partner of the opportunity to connect with the real you.

Perfectionism traps you in a cycle of dissatisfaction, fear, and isolation by tying your self-worth to unrealistic standards. Breaking free from this pattern requires embracing vulnerability, accepting imperfection as a natural part of being human, and allowing your authentic self to be seen by those around you. This openness paves the way for deeper, more fulfilling connections.

Chronic Anxiety

Growing up in a toxic family environment often means living with constant stress and unpredictability, which can lead to chronic anxiety. This type of anxiety becomes deeply ingrained as a survival mechanism, where you remain constantly on edge, anticipating something going wrong. In adulthood, this anxiety can profoundly impact your intimate relationships, leading to persistent worry, overthinking, and the inability to feel secure.

Chronic anxiety in relationships often manifests as a constant sense of dread, where you're continually preoccupied with the fear that someone important to you will leave or that something bad will happen. Even in calm or stable moments, your mind can remain locked in a cycle of "what ifs," focusing on worst-case scenarios that may never materialize. This leaves you emotionally exhausted and disconnected, making it hard to engage fully in the present moment with the people around you.

The roots of this anxiety can often be traced back to the chaotic dynamics of a toxic family. If your caregivers were inconsistent, critical, or emotionally unavailable, you may have learned that relationships are inherently unstable and that security is something fleeting and unreliable. These early experiences create an internalized belief that emotional connection is fragile, and this belief follows you into your adult relationships, often triggering anxiety at the smallest signs of conflict or emotional distance.

Healing from chronic anxiety, especially when it stems from childhood experiences in a toxic family, often requires therapy. Therapy provides a structured and safe space to explore the deep-seated fears and emotional responses that fuel your anxiety. A therapist can help you understand how your early environment shaped your emotional landscape and how these patterns persist into adulthood.

Insecure Attachment Styles
Attachment theory, developed by psychologist John Bowlby, explains how the emotional bonds formed with caregivers in childhood shape our ability to form relationships throughout life. The quality of caregiving you received—whether it was consistent and nurturing or unpredictable and neglectful—plays a crucial role in shaping your attachment style. A secure attachment develops when a caregiver is emotionally available and responsive, creating a sense of safety and trust. However, when a child grows up in a toxic family environment, where caregiving is inconsistent or emotionally absent, insecure attachment styles often emerge.

There are two main types of insecure attachment: anxious and avoidant. Anxious attachment is rooted in a fear of abandonment and a deep need for constant reassurance. If your caregiver was unpredictable—sometimes loving, sometimes distant—you likely learned to cling to them for emotional security, fearing that they could withdraw at any moment. This leads to a heightened sensitivity to rejection and a tendency to become overly dependent on others for validation. In adult relationships, this manifests as anxiety, clinginess, and a need for frequent reassurance from your partner, often out of fear that they may leave you.

Avoidant attachment, on the other hand, develops when caregivers are emotionally unavailable or dismissive of your needs. In response, you may have learned to suppress your emotional needs, relying only on yourself because seeking comfort or connection from others felt unsafe or fruitless. As an adult, you might avoid emotional intimacy, keeping your distance to protect yourself from the potential pain of rejection. This can result in emotional detachment and a reluctance to depend on others, as you've learned to associate closeness with vulnerability and emotional pain.

These attachment styles can create significant challenges in relationships. Anxiously attached individuals often become clingy, seeking constant validation, while individuals with avoidant attachment tend to distance themselves, avoiding vulnerability. This dynamic can lead to a cycle of instability, where one partner feels overwhelmed by the other's neediness, and the other feels emotionally starved or rejected. The result is dissatisfaction on both sides, as both partners struggle to find emotional security.

Understanding your attachment style is an important step toward toxic family healing. By recognizing the patterns shaped by your early caregiving experiences, you can begin to shift how you relate to others consciously. Developing a secure attachment in adulthood is possible, but it requires self-awareness, patience, and, often, the support of a partner who understands these dynamics. Therapy can also be a valuable tool in helping you reframe your understanding of connection and intimacy, allowing you to build healthier, more secure relationships over time.

Low Self-Esteem, Hypersensitivity to Invalidation, and the Fear

of Abandonment

Self-esteem reflects how much you value and appreciate yourself. In a healthy family, children receive consistent support, validation, and encouragement, fostering a strong sense of self-worth. However, in a toxic family environment, where criticism, neglect, or emotional abuse are common, this crucial foundation is undermined. Growing up under such conditions, you may internalize feelings of inadequacy and develop a distorted view of your self-worth.

As a child in a toxic family, you likely experienced relentless criticism, belittling, or the pressure to meet unrealistic expectations. These experiences can teach you that your worth is conditional and that you're constantly falling short. Rather than developing confidence and competence, you may internalize self-doubt and view yourself through a lens of inadequacy. This low self-esteem often carries over into adulthood, especially in your relationships.

In adult relationships, low self-esteem can manifest as a constant need for validation. You may find yourself relying heavily on your partner's opinions or approval, questioning your worth and fearing rejection if you aren't "good enough." This need for validation can create unhealthy dependency, where your sense of self is determined by how others perceive you. Low self-esteem may also lead you to settle for less than you deserve, tolerating mistreatment because you believe you're unworthy of anything better.

Hypersensitivity to invalidation often goes hand-in-hand with low self-esteem. If you grew up in a toxic family where your emotions were dismissed or invalidated, you might have developed a heightened emotional reaction to any form of perceived criticism or neglect. Even small, unintended slights in your adult relationships can feel like significant rejections, reinforcing feelings of worthlessness and inadequacy.

This emotional hypersensitivity can lead to constant self-doubt as you struggle to differentiate between actual rejection and perceived invalidation. You may find yourself seeking constant reassurance from your partner, fearing that even minor misunderstandings mean you're unworthy of affection or that your needs are being dismissed. This hypersensitivity can make relationships emotionally exhausting, as you are always on guard for signs of disapproval or rejection.

The fear of invalidation often ties into a more profound fear of abandonment. If your emotional needs were consistently neglected in childhood, you may have internalized the belief that you are unworthy of care and attention and that abandonment is inevitable. This fear frequently manifests in clingy behaviors, people-pleasing, or an overwhelming need for reassurance in adult relationships. The idea of expressing your true feelings or needs might feel too risky, leading you to suppress them to avoid conflict, rejection, or abandonment.

The fear of abandonment often creates a vicious cycle where you overcompensate in relationships, attempting to control the environment and behaviors of your partner. You might feel as though you must constantly act in ways that please them, much like you did with your toxic family, fearing that a single misstep could result in being left alone. This pressure to be perfect can result in possessiveness, jealousy, and controlling behaviors as you try to prevent any situation that could lead to abandonment. As you struggle with this need for control, the relationship becomes emotionally tense as both partners grapple with the fear that anything could go wrong.

One of the most damaging consequences of this fear is the tendency to hide your authentic self. To avoid conflict or disapproval, you may suppress your true thoughts, desires, and needs, focusing instead on what you believe will keep your partner happy. Over time, this creates a disconnection between who you are and the version of yourself you present in the relationship. This emotional dissonance can lead to resentment, frustration, and emotional exhaustion as you constantly prioritize your partner's needs over your own, losing touch with your identity.

Ironically, the effort to hide your authentic self and avoid conflict often backfires. The constant pressure to be perfect or to avoid any confrontation creates emotional distance. Without authentic communication and vulnerability, misunderstandings and unresolved frustrations accumulate. What starts as an attempt to preserve the relationship can eventually drive you and your partner further apart, as both sides remain disconnected and unsatisfied. The fear of abandonment may lead to the very outcomes you tried so hard to prevent, as the relationship becomes strained by hidden emotions and unmet needs.

To address this deeply ingrained fear of abandonment, you must first acknowledge its origins in your toxic family dynamics and begin the process of unlearning the belief that connection is conditional upon perfection. Part of the healing journey involves embracing your authentic self and trusting that you are worthy of acceptance, even with your flaws. Open communication, setting healthy boundaries, and understanding that no relationship is perfect are essential steps toward breaking free from the cycle of fear and insecurity. Building healthier, more secure relationships requires trusting that you can make mistakes, show your true self, and still be accepted and valued.

In the end, confronting the deep-rooted patterns of low self-esteem, hypersensitivity to invalidation, and fear of abandonment can transform your relationships, allowing you to experience deeper intimacy, emotional security, and genuine connection.

Manipulation and Control

Manipulation is a common tactic in toxic families used to

control behavior and maintain power. As a child, you might have been manipulated through guilt-tripping, emotional blackmail, or gaslighting. These manipulative tactics teach you that affection and approval are conditional and must be earned by conforming to the manipulator's demands. As an adult, you might find yourself either repeating these manipulative behaviors or being drawn to partners who use similar tactics. This creates a cycle of manipulation and control that undermines trust and mutual respect in your relationships.

Neglect and Emotional Abandonment

Neglect, both physical and emotional, is another hallmark of toxic family dynamics. In a neglectful environment, your basic emotional needs for attention, validation, and affection are unmet. This lack of emotional support can lead to feelings of unworthiness and a deep-seated fear of abandonment. As an adult, you might become overly dependent on your partner for emotional validation or fear being left alone, leading to clingy or possessive behaviors that strain the relationship.

Abuse and Trauma

Abuse, whether physical, emotional, or verbal, leaves deep scars that impact your self-esteem and emotional health. Growing up in an abusive environment teaches you to expect mistreatment and disrespect in relationships. As a result, you might tolerate abusive behavior from partners or, conversely, exhibit abusive behaviors yourself. The trauma from past abuse can also cause intense emotional reactions and trigger responses that are disproportionate to the current situation, leading to frequent conflicts and misunderstandings in your relationships.

Inconsistent Caregiving

Inconsistent caregiving creates an unstable and unpredictable environment. When caregivers alternate between loving and neglectful, it creates confusion and insecurity. As a child, you learn to be hypervigilant, constantly on the lookout for changes in mood or behavior to protect yourself. This hypervigilance carries over into adult relationships, where you might become anxious and mistrustful, always expecting the worst from your partner. This constant state of alertness prevents you from fully relaxing and enjoying the relationship.

Lack of Healthy Emotional Support

A toxic family environment often lacks healthy emotional support, leaving you ill-equipped to handle your own emotions and those of others. Without role models who demonstrate healthy emotional expression and regulation, you might struggle with emotional intelligence. This can lead to difficulties in communicating your feelings, managing conflicts, and providing or seeking support in relationships. The result is a relationship fraught with misunderstandings, emotional outbursts, and unresolved issues.

Learned Helplessness

Learned helplessness is a condition where you feel powerless to change your circumstances due to repeated exposure to uncontrollable negative events. In a toxic family, you might have been subjected to unpredictable punishments or arbitrary rules, leading to a sense of helplessness. This learned helplessness can persist into adulthood, causing you to feel trapped in unhealthy relationships without the belief that you can improve your situation. You might tolerate toxic behaviors from your partner, believing that you have no other options.

Fear of Intimacy

Growing up in a toxic family, where emotional closeness might have been associated with pain or rejection, can result in a fear of intimacy. You might find it difficult to trust others and be vulnerable, fearing that emotional closeness will lead to hurt and disappointment. This fear of intimacy can manifest as pushing partners away, avoiding deep emotional connections, or sabotaging relationships when they start to become serious.

Overcoming this fear requires understanding its roots and gradually building trust and emotional resilience.

Unrealistic Expectations and Disappointment

Growing up in a toxic family can instill unrealistic expectations about connection and relationships. You might expect your partner to fulfill all your emotional needs, provide constant reassurance, or behave in unrealistic ways. When these expectations are not met, they can lead to disappointment, resentment, and conflict. Recognizing and adjusting these unrealistic expectations is crucial for building healthier, more realistic relationships.

Communication Breakdown

Effective communication is the foundation of healthy relationships, but toxic family dynamics often disrupt the development of strong communication skills. You may have learned to suppress your true feelings to avoid conflict or rely on passive-aggressive behavior to express your needs indirectly. These patterns can create confusion, misunderstandings, unresolved conflicts, and emotional distance in adult relationships. Overcoming these habits requires learning to communicate openly, honestly, and respectfully. To avoid resentment and foster healthier connections, it is essential to be your authentic self in all intimate relationships, using honest communication and clear boundaries. If you are not true to yourself, your partner will likely disappoint you because they are responding to a version of you that isn't real.

Passive-aggressive communication is another toxic pattern often learned in a toxic family environment. This behavior involves expressing negative feelings indirectly rather than openly addressing them. It can include sulking, giving the silent treatment, making sarcastic remarks, or intentionally failing to fulfill responsibilities.

In relationships, passive-aggressive communication can lead to misunderstandings and unresolved conflicts. Instead of discussing issues openly and honestly, you might resort to subtle digs or withdrawal, leaving your partner confused and hurt. This behavior prevents effective communication and problem-solving, causing ongoing tension and resentment.

In a toxic family, conflict might have been met with aggression, hostility, or punishment, teaching you that it is safer to avoid confrontation altogether. As an adult, this avoidance of conflict can result in suppressed emotions and unresolved issues, which fester and create distance in your relationships.

Avoiding conflict often leads to pretending everything is fine when it is not, refusing to address problems, and sacrificing one's needs to keep the peace. This behavior prevents authentic connection and growth in relationships, as important issues are never discussed or resolved.

Emotional Burnout
Growing up in a toxic family often means being in a constant state of emotional hypervigilance—always on guard to avoid conflict or meet the unrealistic demands of others. This continuous emotional strain can lead to burnout, leaving you feeling exhausted, depleted, and disconnected from your own needs. As a child, you may have learned to prioritize the emotions of others over your own, a pattern that can carry over into adulthood. In adult relationships, this can make it difficult to engage fully, leaving you with little emotional energy to support your partner or maintain a healthy connection.

Toxic family dynamics create an environment where you constantly try to manage others' emotions, often at the expense of your own well-being. Over time, this emotional labor wears you down, leading to burnout. Recognizing the signs—such as chronic fatigue, irritability, and emotional numbness—is crucial.

Rejuvenating your emotional energy by setting boundaries, prioritizing self-care, and seeking support is vital to prevent burnout and maintain fulfilling, healthy relationships.

The Impact of Conditional Love in Toxic Families
Conditional love is a hallmark of toxic family dynamics. In such families, affection and approval are often contingent on meeting specific expectations set by parents or caregivers. For example, a child might receive praise only when they achieve high grades, excel in sports, or conform to the family's expectations. However, when they fall short, they are ignored, criticized, or even punished. This conditional affection teaches the child that love and validation are transactional—that their worth is tied to their performance or behavior rather than being inherent. As a result, they learn to constantly strive for external approval, believing that love must be earned.

In families where conditional love is the norm, the standards for approval may shift frequently, leaving the child in a constant state of confusion and emotional distress. One day, their behavior might meet parental expectations and earn praise, but the next day, the same behavior could be met with indifference or criticism. This inconsistency leaves the child feeling unsure of their value and compels them to suppress their true self in order to avoid rejection. Over time, this conditional dynamic becomes internalized, causing them to believe that they must continuously prove their worth to receive affection—a belief that often persists into adulthood and shapes their intimate relationships.

As adults, individuals who grew up in toxic families may carry these damaging patterns into their relationships. They often believe that affection and approval must be earned through compliance, self-sacrifice, or by meeting their partner's expectations. For example, they might go to great lengths to prioritize their partner's needs over their own, thinking this is the only way to maintain the relationship. They may also be drawn to partners who withhold affection or approval unless certain conditions are met, reinforcing the toxic cycle they experienced in childhood.

In intimate relationships, conditional love can manifest in various ways. A partner might withhold affection, attention, or approval unless specific conditions are met—such as adhering to a certain appearance, agreeing with their opinions, or consistently prioritizing their needs over your own. The recipient of this conditional affection often feels pressure to conform, suppressing their true thoughts and feelings out of fear that any deviation from their partner's expectations will result in withdrawal or rejection. Over time, this dynamic erodes their sense of self and autonomy, leaving them feeling trapped and unfulfilled.

At its most extreme, conditional love can resemble emotional manipulation. A partner may offer affection or validation as a reward when their demands are met but withhold it when they are dissatisfied. This creates a cycle of dependency, where the individual is left constantly striving to meet their partner's conditions, never feeling secure or truly valued in the relationship. This pattern mirrors the toxic family dynamic, where love was conditional upon meeting a caregiver's expectations, and the fear of rejection drove the individual to continually suppress their own needs in favor of maintaining the relationship.

Breaking free from the cycle of conditional love requires recognizing its origins in toxic family dynamics. Understanding how your early experiences shaped your perceptions of affection, self-worth, and relationships is the first step toward healing. In healthy relationships, connection and care are not earned by meeting demands or sacrificing your authenticity; they are given freely and rooted in mutual respect and acceptance. By setting clear boundaries, asserting your own needs, and recognizing that you deserve unconditional acceptance, you can begin to dismantle the destructive patterns of conditional love and cultivate healthier, more secure relationships.

This healing process takes time and often requires deep emotional work. Therapy can be an invaluable resource on this journey, providing a safe space to explore the roots of your relationship patterns and process painful emotions. A skilled therapist can help you develop practical tools for setting healthy boundaries, fostering self-compassion, and rebuilding your sense of self-worth. As you grow in emotional awareness and confidence, you'll be able to break free from the damaging effects of conditional love and embrace relationships that are fulfilling, authentic, and supportive of your true self.

Trying to Fix Others

Growing up in a toxic family environment often forces you to prioritize others' needs above your own as a survival mechanism, usually to avoid conflict or emotional withdrawal. As a child, expressing your true feelings may have led to punishment, anger, or manipulation from those around you, so over time, you learned that keeping the peace was more important than honoring your own desires. This form of self-suppression, where you stifle your true feelings and needs to maintain harmony, can leave you feeling disconnected from your authentic self. You become more concerned with pleasing others than with fulfilling your emotional needs, hindering your personal growth and well-being.

As an adult, this pattern can continue in your relationships. You might constantly prioritize your partner's needs over your own, not because you want to, but because it feels safer. You may fear that asserting your boundaries or expressing your true desires will lead to rejection, conflict, or emotional pain. This often results in people-pleasing behaviors, where you put others' well-being ahead of your own, leading to emotional exhaustion and frustration.

However, trying to "fix" others or manage their emotions is not a sustainable solution. Instead of stepping in to solve problems or soothe every emotional upset, learning to be a mindful observer allows you to witness others' experiences without becoming entangled in their emotional states. Being a mindful observer means offering empathy and support while maintaining your own emotional boundaries and allowing others to take responsibility for their own feelings and reactions.

This shift from "fixing" to "observing" fosters healthier emotional boundaries. You can offer compassion and listen with empathy without the need to solve or control the situation. This approach helps you avoid overstepping into someone else's emotional landscape, allowing both you and your partner to maintain your emotional autonomy. It creates a space for others to process their own emotions while you protect your well-being.

Letting go of the need to fix others can be challenging, particularly if you've been conditioned to take on their emotional burdens. However, stepping back and allowing others the freedom to navigate their emotions fosters healthier relationships. You'll find yourself less emotionally drained and more connected to your authentic self, creating relationships that are balanced and fulfilling. By observing mindfully, you offer support from a place of clarity and strength without losing sight of your own needs, ultimately allowing for deeper, more genuine connections.

This approach to mindful observation helps to avoid emotional enmeshment, where boundaries blur and the needs of one person overshadow the other. Instead, it fosters emotional independence in relationships while preserving empathy. Both you and your partner can experience greater emotional freedom, leading to healthier and more balanced connections where compassion and autonomy coexist.

Reclaiming Your Authentic Self through Self-Care and Boundaries
Healing from toxic family dynamics starts with self-care and

setting healthy boundaries. If your needs were dismissed or invalidated growing up, you may have internalized the belief that your worth is tied to how much you can give to others. This belief can lead to self-sacrifice, people-pleasing, and neglecting your own emotional needs. To heal, it's crucial to recognize that caring for your own well-being is not only valid but necessary for creating balanced relationships.

Setting boundaries helps you reconnect with your authentic self and prioritize self-care. This process involves taking care of your mental, emotional, and physical health and learning to say "no" when your boundaries are crossed. By placing your well-being at the center of your life, you break free from the toxic patterns of dependency, fear of abandonment, and constant self-sacrifice. In doing so, you build reciprocal and fulfilling relationships where both your true self and emotional needs are valued.

Chapter 1 Conclusion

The lasting effects of growing up in a toxic family can feel overwhelming, but by recognizing and confronting these emotional scars, you're already on the path to healing. From a lack of trust and emotional instability to perfectionism, anxiety, fear of abandonment, and unhealthy attachment styles, these patterns were your survival mechanisms in a toxic environment. However, they no longer serve you in your adult relationships. The fact that you're here, reflecting on these behaviors, shows that you're ready to take control of your healing journey, and that's a powerful first step.

Healing from these deep wounds begins with self-awareness. By understanding the roots of your insecurities, anxiety, and emotional patterns, you gain the clarity needed to begin unlearning them. You've been shaped by the unpredictable nature of your toxic family—constantly adapting to emotional chaos, struggling to feel worthy, and learning to fear vulnerability. But here's the truth: You don't have to remain stuck in those patterns. Your past does not have to dictate your future.

It's important to acknowledge that this journey will take time, but it is one worth taking. As you move forward, you'll uncover the secrets to breaking free from the toxic dynamics that have held you back. You'll learn how to foster trust, emotional stability, and genuine intimacy in your relationships. You'll replace perfectionism with self-acceptance, embrace vulnerability as a strength, and discover that true emotional connection is built on honesty, not fear. The sense of powerlessness and helplessness that haunted you can be transformed into self-confidence and emotional resilience.

By addressing low self-esteem and hypersensitivity to invalidation, you'll begin to see that your worth is not defined by others' approval or criticism. You'll break free from the cycle of seeking external validation and begin to trust in your own value. This shift will open the door to healthier, more balanced relationships—where your authentic self is honored and where your emotional needs are met. You'll no longer be defined by the manipulative control, neglect, or abandonment you endured as a child. Instead, you'll learn how to reclaim your personal power, set healthy boundaries, and protect your emotional well-being.

Over time, you'll recognize the unhealthy attachment styles you may have developed—whether anxious or avoidant—and learn to cultivate a secure attachment. This will allow you to connect more deeply with your partner without fear of rejection or abandonment. You'll also confront the unrealistic expectations and communication breakdowns that stem from your toxic upbringing, empowering you to express yourself openly and honestly in your relationships. These skills will not only strengthen your intimate connections but also help you feel more at ease within yourself.

As you continue this healing journey, you'll uncover the secrets to overcoming the patterns that have kept you stuck. You'll learn how to let go of self-sacrifice, stop people-pleasing, and start prioritizing your emotional needs. The emotional wounds you've carried for so long can finally begin to heal as you break free from manipulation, conditional approval, and the need to "fix" others. Instead, you'll focus on reclaiming your authentic self and building relationships that are rooted in mutual respect, emotional freedom, and unwavering trust.

This journey is about rediscovering who you are beneath the scars and stepping into a life where the dynamics of your past no longer control you. You'll learn to protect your emotional energy, create healthier boundaries, and cultivate self-respect, all while allowing others to see and appreciate your true self. The road may not always be easy, but the transformation is worth it.

By continuing on this path, you'll uncover the secrets to building healthy, intimate relationships and reclaiming the emotional freedom you deserve. Healing from a toxic family is possible, and with each step forward, you're moving closer to the fulfilling, authentic life that has always been waiting for you. The future is yours to create, one filled with deeper connections, healthier relationships, and, most importantly, self-love.

2. Transcending Automatic Defense Mechanisms in Relationships

Automatic defense mechanisms are deeply ingrained survival strategies that often originate in toxic family environments. When growing up in a household where emotional or psychological safety is compromised, the brain learns to respond quickly to perceived threats, even in situations where danger may not exist. These mechanisms, such as avoidance, numbing, or people-pleasing, were essential during childhood to protect against harm and maintain a sense of control.

However, as adults, these deeply embedded patterns often resurface in intimate relationships, unconsciously shaping how we interact with loved ones. While once protective, these automatic responses can hinder emotional connection, trust, and vulnerability, perpetuating cycles of emotional distance and conflict. Transcending these defenses is essential for building healthy, lasting relationships free from the scars of the past.

Growing up in a toxic family environment, I learned to rely on automatic defense mechanisms to protect myself from emotional harm. In a household where criticism and emotional invalidation were constants, I developed a heightened sense of vigilance, always anticipating the next outburst or emotional wound. As a child, this hyper-awareness helped me navigate an unpredictable world—it became a survival strategy. I also became a people-pleaser, bending over backward to meet others' expectations, hoping that it would shield me from criticism or rejection. These defense mechanisms served me well in the moment, allowing me to maintain some semblance of control over an otherwise chaotic environment.

However, as I entered adult relationships, these same survival strategies began to backfire. When conflict arose, I would either get angry and confrontational—instinctively moving into "fight" mode—or I would shut down completely, retreating into silence as my "flight" response took over. These reactions were automatic, deeply rooted in my childhood experiences of needing to defend myself emotionally or mentally escape when things got too painful. I often didn't realize that by reacting this way, I was pushing my partner away and creating emotional distance, even in moments where connection and understanding were possible. My people-pleasing tendencies also persisted—I often prioritized my partner's needs, even when it meant sacrificing my own well-being, repeating a pattern deeply ingrained from childhood.

Transcending these automatic defense mechanisms has been a slow, deliberate process. I've had to learn to recognize when my defenses are triggered, stepping back to assess whether the threat is real or simply a residue of my past. In moments of conflict, I remind myself that my anger or urge to withdraw doesn't necessarily reflect the present reality. By gradually letting go of the instinct to fight or flee, I've started to build more authentic connections in my relationships—ones grounded in trust and openness rather than fear and avoidance. This journey hasn't been easy, but breaking free from these patterns has allowed me to experience deeper emotional connections and create a healthier foundation for my relationships.

These automatic defense mechanisms, while essential for survival in a toxic family environment, often become roadblocks to healthy, fulfilling relationships as adults. The fight or flight responses that helped me navigate the unpredictability of my childhood no longer serve the same purpose in adult relationships. Instead, they create emotional disconnection, misunderstandings, and strain, pushing away the very intimacy I long for. The tendency to either react with anger or shut down completely prevents me from engaging in open, honest communication and from understanding the real needs of my partner.

What once protected me from emotional harm now acts as a barrier to the deep connection and trust that are essential for a healthy relationship. The people-pleasing tendencies I developed reinforce a pattern of sacrificing my own well-being to avoid conflict or rejection, ultimately leading to resentment and emotional exhaustion. These deeply ingrained survival mechanisms, though automatic and subconscious, are no longer necessary or helpful in the context of adult relationships.

Recognizing and working to transcend these defense mechanisms is crucial for breaking free from the unhealthy patterns of the past. By stepping back and assessing whether my reactions are rooted in old wounds rather than present realities, I've learned to navigate conflict with more clarity and compassion. Building relationships on trust and openness, rather than fear and avoidance, has become the foundation for healthier, more fulfilling connections. Though the journey is challenging, each step away from these automatic defenses brings me closer to authentic, meaningful relationships.

Understanding these defense mechanisms, how they are triggered in your life, and how you react to stressful situations in your adult intimate relationships is crucial for anyone seeking to break free from the toxic family patterns of their past. By recognizing how these responses manifest in your relationships—whether through aggression, withdrawal, emotional numbness, or people-pleasing —you can begin to address and transform them.

Recognizing when your defense mechanisms are triggered allows you to step back and assess whether the perceived threat is real or just a remnant of past trauma. This self-awareness is the first step toward changing how you react in stressful situations. Instead of falling into old patterns of anger or avoidance, you can begin to choose healthier responses that promote openness and vulnerability. Over time, this will help you build stronger, more genuine connections based on trust rather than fear or self-protection.

This chapter will guide you through the most common defense mechanisms, illustrating how they operate and offering strategies for overcoming their negative impact. By learning to transcend these automatic responses, you can break the cycle of toxic patterns and create a healthier, more fulfilling relationship dynamic.

Fight Response: Aggression, Confrontation, Defensiveness

The fight response is a deeply rooted survival mechanism that often manifests in adult relationships as aggression, confrontation, and defensiveness. For those who grew up in toxic family environments—where conflict was ever-present or where they had to battle to have their needs met—this response can become a habitual way of interacting with others. While it may have been essential for survival in a hostile or neglectful environment, this instinctual reaction can be highly detrimental when carried into adult relationships, where it often escalates minor disagreements into major conflicts and fosters a hostile atmosphere.

Origins and the Brain's Role in the Fight Response

The fight response originates from the brain's instinctual need to protect itself from perceived threats. In a toxic family environment, where verbal, emotional, or physical harm was a constant risk, the brain—particularly the amygdala—becomes hyper-alert to signs of danger. The amygdala, responsible for processing emotions like fear and anger, plays a central role in the body's fight-or-flight response. When triggered, the amygdala overrides the prefrontal cortex, the part of the brain responsible for rational thinking, emotional regulation, and decision-making. This override mechanism diminishes feelings of empathy and connection as the brain shifts into survival mode, prioritizing self-defense over emotional engagement.

In such a state, even minor conflicts or disagreements can be perceived as serious threats, leading to an automatic, aggressive response. This response may have been necessary to ensure one's voice was heard or boundaries were respected in a chaotic environment. However, in adult relationships, where safety and mutual respect are ideally the norm, this heightened response is not only unnecessary but also harmful. It can lead to an escalation of conflicts, where instead of resolving issues through calm discussion, interactions quickly spiral into heated arguments or even physical confrontations.

The Fight Response in Relationships
In adult relationships, the fight response often reveals itself through several behaviors that can damage the foundation of trust and intimacy. One common manifestation is aggression, which can be verbal, such as yelling, name-calling, or making hurtful comments, or physical, including intimidating gestures or actual violence. This aggression stems from the brain's misinterpretation of the situation as dangerous, prompting an all-out defense.

Another manifestation is extreme confrontation. Individuals with a strong fight response may approach every disagreement as a battle that must be won rather than as an opportunity to understand and resolve differences. This confrontational approach often leaves their partner feeling attacked, defensive, and misunderstood, which only serves to deepen the conflict.

Defensiveness is another key aspect of the fight response. When someone is defensive, they react to feedback or perceived criticism by immediately justifying their actions, denying any wrongdoing, or turning the blame back on the other person. This shuts down open communication and prevents any genuine understanding or resolution from occurring. For example, if a partner expresses feelings of hurt, the defensive individual might respond with, "It's not my fault," or "You're just being too sensitive," rather than addressing the concern with empathy and a willingness to understand.

Breaking the Cycle of the Fight Response

Recognizing the fight response as an automatic defense mechanism rooted in survival instincts is the first step toward breaking its hold on your relationships. Understanding that these aggressive behaviors are not a true reflection of your feelings but rather a conditioned response to perceived threats can help you begin to change these patterns.

The journey to overcoming the fight response begins with self-awareness. Start by paying close attention to how you react during conflicts. Notice when you feel the urge to become aggressive, confrontational, or defensive. This awareness allows you to pause before acting on these impulses, giving you the chance to choose a more constructive and positive response.

Active listening is another crucial skill in managing the fight response. Instead of immediately reacting to your partner's words, take the time to listen fully and understand their perspective. Reflect on what you've heard and ask clarifying questions if needed. This approach not only helps to de-escalate potentially tense situations but also demonstrates to your partner that you value their feelings and opinions.

Healthy communication is key to replacing aggressive responses with more effective interactions. Work on expressing your thoughts and feelings calmly and assertively, using "I" statements to convey your emotions without blaming or accusing your partner. For instance, instead of saying, "You never listen to me," you could say, "I feel unheard when I'm interrupted during our conversations." This shift in language fosters a more open and less confrontational dialogue.

If anger frequently fuels your fight response, it's important to explore ways to manage this emotion constructively. Techniques such as deep breathing, taking a moment to cool down, or engaging in physical exercise can help you calm down before addressing the issue at hand. Over time, these practices can reduce the intensity of your fight response and help you approach conflict with greater clarity and empathy.

Transforming the fight response into more constructive behaviors takes time and practice. However, by committing to this process, you can create a more peaceful and supportive relationship dynamic. As you learn to respond to conflicts with calmness and empathy, you'll likely find that your relationships become more fulfilling, with greater mutual understanding and respect. Over time, the fight response can be replaced with healthier ways of communicating and connecting, leading to deeper emotional intimacy and stronger, more resilient relationships.

Flight Response: Avoidance, Withdrawal, Escapism

In relationships, the flight response is a deeply ingrained survival mechanism that manifests as a need to escape from situations that feel threatening or overwhelming. This behavior, which often develops in response to toxic family dynamics, can significantly impact emotional intimacy and connection in adult relationships. For many, the instinct to flee—whether physically, emotionally, or mentally—was learned in environments where confrontation or emotional expression was met with hostility. As adults, these learned behaviors can take various forms, including avoidance, withdrawal, or escapism, each contributing to the gradual erosion of a relationship's foundation.

The Brain's Role in the Flight Response

The brain plays a crucial role in triggering the flight response. Specifically, the amygdala—the brain's center for processing emotions like fear—becomes hyperactive when it perceives a threat. This reaction prompts the brain to switch into "survival mode," where the primary objective is self-preservation. In this state, the brain seeks to protect you by avoiding perceived danger, even if that danger is not real but rather a residual effect of past experiences. The brain's response can cause you to interpret neutral or even positive interactions as potentially harmful, leading you to pull away from your partner.

The Flight Response in Relationships

In a relationship, the flight response often shows up as avoidance, withdrawal, and escapism. Avoidance might involve steering clear of difficult conversations, shying away from intimacy, or refusing to acknowledge underlying issues that need addressing. For instance, you might consistently avoid discussions about your partner's concerns, hoping that by doing so, the issue will simply go away. However, this only leads to unresolved tensions, quietly undermining the relationship.

Withdrawal is another common expression of the flight response. Here, you may emotionally distance yourself from your partner, reducing communication, physical affection, or even daily interactions. Over time, this withdrawal can create a significant gap between partners, as one becomes increasingly disconnected while the other feels abandoned and confused. The belief that pulling back will protect you from potential hurt often deepens the emotional chasm instead.

Escapism takes this a step further by involving a physical

or mental removal from the relationship. You might immerse yourself in work, hobbies, or even excessive social media use to avoid confronting relationship issues. While this may provide temporary relief, it ultimately exacerbates emotional distance and leaves critical problems unaddressed. For example, spending more time at the office or engaging in solitary activities might serve as an escape from the discomfort of emotional closeness, inadvertently sending the message that your partner's needs and the relationship itself are not priorities.

Breaking Free from the Flight Response
Breaking free from the flight response requires a conscious effort to understand and counteract these deeply ingrained behaviors. Recognizing that your brain is operating in survival mode is the first step in challenging these instincts. It's important to realize that the threats your brain perceives are often echoes of past experiences rather than present realities. By bringing awareness to these automatic responses, you can begin to choose healthier, more constructive ways of engaging with your partner.

Therapeutic Strategies for Overcoming the Flight Response
Therapeutic strategies, such as mindfulness practices and cognitive-behavioral therapy (CBT), are not just effective but also empowering tools in addressing the flight response. They can help you stay present in the moment, recognize when you're beginning to retreat, and provide you with the tools to remain engaged. CBT, in particular, is a powerful approach that can reframe negative thought patterns and replace avoidance with more adaptive behaviors, giving you the power to take control of your responses.

It's important to understand that dismantling the flight response is a gradual process. By gradually confronting the discomfort that triggers the flight response, you can begin to dismantle the walls that have built up over time. This process won't happen overnight, but with persistence and support, it's possible to transform the flight response from a barrier into a bridge that fosters deeper connection and intimacy in your relationships.

Freeze Response: Numbing, Shutting Down, Dissociation

The freeze response is a powerful and often misunderstood defense mechanism that individuals use to protect themselves from overwhelming stress, conflict, or emotional pain. Unlike the fight or flight responses, which involve active attempts to confront or escape a threat, the freeze response is characterized by a profound withdrawal from the situation. This withdrawal can manifest as emotional numbing, shutting down, or even dissociation, all of which create significant barriers to emotional intimacy and healthy communication within relationships.

The Brain's Role in the Freeze Response
The freeze response is deeply rooted in the brain's survival mechanisms. When faced with a situation where neither fighting nor fleeing seems possible, the brain triggers the freeze response as a final line of defense. This reaction is primarily governed by the amygdala and the hypothalamus—regions of the brain responsible for processing emotions and detecting threats. When these areas are activated, the brain essentially tells the body to "play dead" in an attempt to avoid further harm.

During this state, the brain's priority shifts from connection and interaction to self-preservation. The amygdala, in particular, sends signals that cause the body to become still, the mind to detach, and emotions to shut down. This automatic response can create a psychological distance between you and your partner, making it difficult to engage in meaningful conversations or emotional exchanges.

The Freeze Response in Relationships
In relationships, the freeze response can take on several forms, each of which can disrupt the flow of healthy communication

and emotional intimacy. Emotional numbing is one of the most common manifestations, where an individual becomes unresponsive to their partner's emotions and needs. This numbing can make it seem as though the person doesn't care, even when that's far from the truth. Instead, it's a sign that the individual is overwhelmed and has temporarily shut down emotionally to cope.

Shutting down is another expression of the freeze response. In moments of intense stress or conflict, an individual might withdraw completely, becoming silent and distant. This withdrawal can be frustrating and hurtful to the partner who is trying to communicate or resolve an issue. The emotional and physical distance created by shutting down prevents any meaningful resolution from taking place, often leading to misunderstandings and unresolved tension.

Dissociation is perhaps the most extreme form of the freeze response. In this state, an individual may feel disconnected from their own emotions, body, or even reality. They might describe feeling as though they are watching the situation from outside their body, unable to engage or respond. This detachment is the brain's way of protecting the individual from trauma or emotional pain, but it also creates a significant barrier to connection and intimacy. Partners may feel confused, hurt, and helpless as they try to reach someone who seems unreachable.

Breaking the Freeze Response Cycle
Breaking free from the freeze response is a challenging but crucial step toward building healthier relationships. This process begins with self-compassion—understanding that the freeze response is an automatic reaction that developed as a means of survival. Recognizing this can help reduce feelings of shame or guilt and allow for a more compassionate approach to healing.

Therapy can be incredibly beneficial in addressing the freeze response. A therapist can help you explore the root causes of this behavior, often tracing it back to early experiences of trauma or neglect. Through therapy, you can begin to process these past experiences, allowing you to move beyond them and develop healthier coping mechanisms.

Mindfulness practices are also powerful tools for overcoming the freeze response. Techniques such as deep breathing, meditation, and body scanning can help you stay present in the moment, reducing the likelihood of dissociation or emotional numbing. By grounding yourself in the present, you can start to re-engage with your emotions and your partner in a more meaningful way.

Grounding techniques are particularly useful when you feel the freeze response beginning to take hold. These techniques, which might include focusing on your senses or physically connecting with your surroundings, can help bring you back into your body and the present moment. Over time, practicing these techniques can help you build resilience, enabling you to face emotional challenges without resorting to withdrawal or dissociation.

By understanding and addressing the freeze response, you can begin to dismantle the barriers it creates in your relationships. With patience, self-compassion, and proactive effort, it's possible to break the cycle of numbing, shutting down, and dissociation. This process will open the door to deeper emotional connections and healthier, more fulfilling relationships.

Fawn Response: People-Pleasing, Compliance, Caretaking

The fawn response is a deeply ingrained survival mechanism that many people unknowingly carry into their adult relationships. It manifests in behaviors like people-pleasing, excessive compliance, and taking on a caretaking role, often at the expense of one's own needs and well-being. For those who have grown up in toxic family environments, these behaviors are not just habits—they are automatic responses rooted in an unconscious need to avoid conflict and gain approval.

While the fawn response may have served as a protective strategy during childhood, ensuring safety in an unpredictable environment, it can be detrimental in adult relationships, leading to emotional exhaustion, a loss of identity, and a cycle of self-neglect.

The Brain's Role in the Fawn Response

At the core of the fawn response is the brain's instinctual drive to protect itself from perceived threats. When the brain detects potential conflict or disapproval, it triggers a series of automatic reactions aimed at mitigating danger. For someone who has been conditioned to see confrontation or rejection as threats, the brain's default response may be to comply, please, or caretake excessively. This is the brain's way of ensuring safety by neutralizing the perceived threat. In essence, the brain tells the individual that to avoid conflict and maintain relationships, they must put others' needs above their own.

However, while these behaviors may have kept peace in a toxic family environment, they can create significant barriers to genuine intimacy and mutual respect in adult relationships. The brain's automatic response to perceive others as potential threats or to assume that approval must be earned through self-sacrifice becomes a significant obstacle to forming balanced, healthy connections.

The Fawn Response in Relationships

In adult relationships, the fawn response often manifests as people-pleasing behaviors. This can lead to a dynamic where one partner gives endlessly, sacrificing their own needs and desires in an attempt to keep the relationship stable. Unfortunately, this can result in relationships that are one-sided, where the fawning individual is consistently giving without receiving the same level of care or consideration in return. Over time, this imbalance can erode the fawning individual's sense of self-worth. They may begin to feel that their value is tied solely to their ability to please others, leading to emotional burnout and a deep sense of inadequacy.

This cycle of self-neglect and dependency perpetuates the very insecurity that drives the fawn response in the first place. The more an individual fawns, the more they reinforce the belief that they are not enough unless they are giving of themselves constantly. This not only harms their self-esteem but also prevents the development of a truly reciprocal and fulfilling relationship.

Breaking Free from the Fawn Response
Breaking free from the fawn response begins with recognition and self-awareness. Understanding that these behaviors are automatic and rooted in past survival strategies is the first step toward change. Affirming your own worth, independent of others' approval, is crucial in this process. It's important to realize that your value does not depend on how much you can do for others or how well you can avoid conflict.

Setting boundaries is a key part of overcoming the fawn response. This involves learning to say "no" when something doesn't align with your needs or values and understanding that doing so does not diminish your worth or jeopardize your relationships. Boundaries help to create a more balanced dynamic in relationships, where both partners' needs are respected and met.
Practicing self-compassion is also essential. This means treating yourself with the same kindness and understanding that you would offer to a friend. Recognize that it's okay to have needs and that those needs are just as important as anyone else's. Self-compassion can help you rebuild your sense of self-worth and break the cycle of self-neglect.

For many, seeking therapeutic support can be incredibly helpful in this journey. Therapy provides a safe space to explore the root causes of the fawn response and develop healthier ways of interacting with others. Techniques such as mindfulness and assertiveness training can be particularly effective in transforming the fawn response into a more balanced and self-respecting way of engaging with the world.

By understanding and addressing the fawn response, you can begin to reclaim your identity and build relationships grounded in mutual respect and authenticity. This process may take time, but with patience and effort, it is entirely possible to move beyond people-pleasing and create a life where your needs and well-being are valued equally alongside those of others.

Hypervigilance: Constant Alertness, Over-Analysis, Exaggerated Startle Response

Hypervigilance is a state of heightened alertness in which an individual is constantly on guard, scanning their environment for potential threats. This perpetual state of readiness is often a deeply ingrained survival mechanism developed in response to early life trauma or toxic environments. While hypervigilance may have once served as a crucial means of protection, it can become a significant barrier to emotional intimacy, trust, and overall well-being in adult relationships.

The Brain's Role in Hypervigilance

The brain plays a central role in hypervigilance, primarily driven by the amygdala—the brain's alarm system for detecting threats. When someone has experienced trauma or prolonged stress, particularly in a toxic family environment, the amygdala becomes hyperactive. It begins to send constant signals that the person is under threat, even in situations that are objectively safe. This overactivation creates a state of chronic anxiety, where the brain is always on high alert, anticipating danger where there may be none.

This heightened state is not just about being cautious; it's an automatic, often unconscious response that can severely disrupt one's ability to relax and engage meaningfully with others. The brain, conditioned by past experiences, misinterprets benign situations as potential threats, leading to responses that are out of proportion to the actual circumstances. In relationships, this means that an offhand comment, a slight change in tone, or even a delay in communication can be perceived as signs of impending conflict or rejection.

Hypervigilance in Relationships

Hypervigilance manifests in several ways within relationships, each contributing to a cycle of anxiety, mistrust, and emotional distance. One of the most common manifestations is constant alertness. Individuals in this state are always on the lookout for signs of trouble, whether it's a subtle shift in their partner's behavior, a missed text, or a change in routine. This constant scanning for threats can create a tense atmosphere, where the hypervigilant person is never fully present or relaxed, always expecting the worst.

Over-analysis is another hallmark of hypervigilance. Those who struggle with this condition tend to dissect every interaction, searching for hidden meanings or potential problems. Conversations are replayed and scrutinized, with every word and gesture weighed for possible threats. This overthinking can lead to misunderstandings, as the hypervigilant person may jump to negative conclusions, even when there is no factual basis for them. This behavior can strain relationships, as the partner may feel unfairly accused or scrutinized, leading to frustration and emotional withdrawal.

The exaggerated startle response is also common among those experiencing hypervigilance. Sudden noises, unexpected touch, or any abrupt changes in the environment can trigger an intense reaction far beyond what the situation warrants. This heightened sensitivity can make the person seem jumpy or overly reactive, adding to the stress in the relationship. Over time, this exaggerated response can create a dynamic where the partner feels like they are walking on eggshells, unsure of what might trigger the next overreaction.

Breaking the Cycle of Hypervigilance
Breaking free from hypervigilance is not easy, but it is possible with self-awareness, deliberate effort, and supportive practices. The first step is recognizing when hypervigilance is taking over. This awareness allows you to pause and assess whether the perceived threat is real or a product of your brain's automatic response. Mindfulness practices can be particularly helpful here, as they encourage staying present and observing your thoughts and feelings without judgment. By grounding yourself in the present moment, you can begin to challenge the automatic thoughts that fuel hypervigilance.

Cognitive restructuring is another powerful tool for addressing hypervigilance. This involves actively challenging the negative thought patterns that contribute to your heightened state of alertness. When you find yourself jumping to conclusions or assuming the worst, take a step back and ask yourself whether there is concrete evidence to support those thoughts. Over time, this practice can help rewire your brain to respond more calmly and rationally to potential triggers.

In addition to these cognitive strategies, relaxation techniques can help reduce the physiological symptoms of hypervigilance. Deep breathing exercises, progressive muscle relaxation, and other stress-reduction methods can calm the nervous system, making it easier to shift from a state of constant alertness to one of peace and connection. These techniques help to deactivate the amygdala's alarm system, allowing you to engage more fully with your partner without the interference of fear and anxiety.

Open communication with your partner is also crucial in overcoming hypervigilance. By discussing your experiences and triggers, you can work together to create an environment of safety and understanding. This might involve setting boundaries, agreeing on ways to handle conflict, or simply being more attuned to each other's emotional needs. Building trust takes time, but with consistent effort, it is possible to create a relationship where both partners feel secure and connected.

While hypervigilance may have once been a necessary survival mechanism, it can be transformed into healthier ways of relating to others. Through self-awareness, cognitive restructuring, relaxation techniques, and open communication, you can break the cycle of hypervigilance and foster deeper, more trusting relationships.

Perfectionism: High Standards, Overachievement, Fear of Failure

Perfectionism is a defense mechanism characterized by setting excessively high standards, often accompanied by an unrelenting drive to meet these expectations. Rooted in a deep fear of failure, perfectionism is driven by the belief that only flawless performance will earn validation and approval. While this pursuit of perfection may appear admirable on the surface, it often leads to chronic dissatisfaction, anxiety, and significant strain on relationships. The constant pressure to achieve can create emotional distance, as perfectionists may struggle with vulnerability and openness, fearing judgment or rejection if they fall short.

The Brain's Role in Perfectionism

Perfectionism is not just a personality trait; it is a deeply ingrained response driven by the brain's automatic mechanisms. For those who grew up in environments where worth was consistently tied to achievements, the brain learned to equate any potential failure with danger. This creates a state of hyper-vigilance, where the individual constantly strives for perfection as a means of self-preservation. The brain, in its effort to protect, becomes fixated on avoiding mistakes, often at the expense of emotional well-being and relational harmony.

This relentless pursuit of flawlessness is the brain's way of ensuring that one is never vulnerable to criticism, rejection, or abandonment. However, this drive for perfection can become all-consuming, leading to a cycle of stress and burnout. The perfectionist's brain is always on high alert, scanning for potential errors or imperfections, creating a constant state of tension and anxiety.

Perfectionism in Relationships

Perfectionism can create significant imbalances in relationships. The perfectionist's need to achieve often takes precedence over the relationship itself, leading to emotional neglect and distance. Partners of perfectionists may feel as though they are secondary to the perfectionist's ambitions, resulting in feelings of inadequacy, resentment, and emotional disconnection.

The perfectionist may also project their high standards onto their partner, expecting them to meet unrealistic expectations. This can lead to a dynamic where the partner feels constantly judged or criticized, creating tension and eroding trust. The relationship becomes less about mutual support and connection and more about living up to an unattainable ideal.

The psychological toll of perfectionism is profound. The perfectionist is often caught in a cycle of relentless self-criticism, where nothing is ever good enough. This can erode self-esteem and lead to a deep sense of unworthiness, as the individual feels they are never able to live up to their own expectations. The pressure to be perfect can also lead to procrastination and avoidance, as the fear of failure becomes so overwhelming that it paralyzes action.

Overcoming Perfectionism and Embracing Imperfection
Overcoming perfectionism involves a fundamental shift in mindset. It requires challenging the belief that worth is tied to achievements and learning to embrace imperfection as a natural and valuable part of life. This transformation begins with self-compassion—recognizing that it is okay to make mistakes and that these imperfections do not diminish one's value or worth.

Practicing self-compassion allows individuals to break free from the relentless pursuit of perfection and begin to appreciate effort and progress rather than just outcomes. Setting realistic and attainable goals is also crucial in this process. By focusing on growth and learning rather than perfection, individuals can begin to shift their perspective from one of constant self-criticism to one of self-acceptance.

Open communication is essential in relationships affected by perfectionism. Sharing struggles with perfectionism with a partner can create a supportive environment where both individuals can work together to overcome these challenges. By acknowledging vulnerabilities and seeking mutual understanding, couples can build a relationship based on acceptance, trust, and mutual respect rather than on the pressure to be perfect.

Overcoming perfectionism is not about lowering standards or giving up on goals; it is about finding a healthier, more balanced approach to life and relationships. By embracing imperfection and fostering authentic connections, individuals can break free from the constraints of perfectionism and build a life that is both fulfilling and emotionally rich.

Emotional Suppression: Hiding

Feelings, Bottling Up Emotions

Emotional suppression is a defense mechanism where individuals hide their true feelings or bottle up emotions to avoid vulnerability. This behavior often stems from a fear of being judged, rejected, or hurt, particularly if expressing emotions was met with negative consequences in the past. While it may have been a necessary survival tactic in toxic family environments, emotional suppression can create significant barriers to connection in relationships. When emotions are consistently suppressed, it becomes difficult to engage fully with your partner, leading to misunderstandings, emotional distance, and a lack of intimacy.

The Brain's Role in Emotional Suppression and the Need for Connection
The brain plays a critical role in emotional suppression. When it perceives emotional expression as a potential threat—based on past experiences where vulnerability led to harm or rejection—it activates automatic mechanisms designed to protect you. These mechanisms often involve shutting down emotional responses to maintain control and avoid pain. As a result, your brain may start viewing others, even those closest to you, as potential threats, leading to further emotional withdrawal.

When your brain is in fight-or-flight mode, the frontal lobe deprioritizes connection and emotional closeness, focusing instead on survival. This can cause those around you to appear as adversaries, triggering a search for validation and connection that becomes increasingly difficult to satisfy. The automatic suppression of emotions not only inhibits the natural expression of feelings necessary for building and maintaining healthy relationships but also distorts your perceptions and interactions, making it harder to establish fulfilling connections.

Understanding this process is crucial. By recognizing how your brain influences your behavior, you can start addressing these automatic responses. Reprogramming your brain to prioritize connection, even in moments of stress, is essential for fostering healthier, more resilient relationships. This involves actively working to create new neural pathways that encourage openness, trust, and emotional expression rather than retreating into old, protective behaviors.

Impact on Relationships

Consistently hiding feelings or bottling up emotions makes it nearly impossible for your partner to truly know you, creating a sense of distance and disconnection. Your partner may sense that something is wrong but feel powerless to address it because you are not openly sharing your thoughts or feelings. Over time, this emotional gap can widen, leading to misunderstandings, resentment, and a sense of isolation within the relationship.

Moreover, the burden of unexpressed emotions doesn't simply vanish—it accumulates. The energy required to suppress these feelings can lead to sudden emotional outbursts, often triggered by minor incidents. These outbursts may seem disproportionate to the situation, but they are actually the release of pent-up emotions that have been bottled up for too long. Such incidents can catch both you and your partner off guard, leading to further strain and conflict.

In addition to these outbursts, chronic emotional suppression can also manifest in physical health issues. The stress of continually holding back emotions can lead to anxiety, depression, digestive problems, and even cardiovascular issues. This toll on your overall well-being makes it even more challenging to maintain a healthy relationship.

Breaking the Cycle of Emotional Suppression

Breaking free from the cycle of emotional suppression is essential for fostering intimacy and trust in your relationships. The first step is recognizing that this pattern exists and understanding that it was likely developed as a protective mechanism in response to past experiences. Acknowledging that these behaviors, while once useful, are now hindering your ability to connect with others is crucial for making positive changes.

Learning to express your emotions in a healthy way is the next step. This doesn't mean you have to share every feeling immediately, but it's about finding safe spaces where you can begin to explore and express your emotions without fear of judgment or rejection. Therapy, journaling, and mindfulness practices can be valuable tools in this process, helping you reconnect with your emotions and learn to express them constructively. These practices also help reprogram your brain to see vulnerability not as a threat but as a pathway to deeper connection.

Building emotional resilience is another critical component of overcoming emotional suppression. By gradually allowing yourself to experience and express a broader range of emotions, you strengthen your ability to handle emotional challenges without resorting to suppression. This resilience allows you to engage more fully with your partner, creating a relationship dynamic that is open, honest, and emotionally fulfilling.

Emotional suppression and the brain's role in automatic defense mechanisms are deeply intertwined. Understanding and addressing these issues is critical for breaking free from the patterns that have held you back. By learning to express emotions healthily and reprogramming your brain to prioritize connection, you can build relationships that are truly connected, supportive, and fulfilling.

Strategies to Address Automatic Defense Mechanisms

Addressing automatic defense mechanisms requires a comprehensive approach that begins with self-awareness, emotional regulation, and resilience. These deeply ingrained patterns, which often develop in response to toxic family environments, can be transformed into healthier coping mechanisms with intentional practice and dedication.

Recognize and Interrupt Automatic Responses

The first step in managing automatic defense mechanisms is to recognize when they are occurring. This involves being attuned to your emotional and physical reactions in different situations. Mindfulness practices play a crucial role here, as they encourage you to stay present and observe your thoughts and feelings without judgment. By practicing mindfulness, you become more aware of your automatic responses as they occur, which gives you the power to interrupt them before they escalate.

In addition to mindfulness, self-reflection is a valuable tool for identifying these patterns. Regular journaling about your interactions and emotions can provide insights into the triggers and underlying causes of your automatic responses. Understanding these triggers allows you to anticipate and manage your reactions more effectively.

Body awareness is another key aspect of recognizing automatic responses. By paying attention to physical sensations, such as a tightening in your chest or a clenching of your jaw, you can detect the onset of a fight or flight response. This awareness gives you the opportunity to take steps to calm yourself before the response fully takes hold. Techniques such as progressive muscle relaxation, where you tense and then relax different muscle groups, can help you become more attuned to your body's signals.

Develop Healthier Coping Mechanisms

Once you've identified your automatic responses, the next step is to replace them with healthier coping mechanisms. Deep breathing exercises are highly effective in calming the nervous system and reducing the intensity of these responses. By practicing slow, deep breaths—inhale for a count of four, hold for a count of four, and exhale for a count of four—you can activate your parasympathetic nervous system, which helps to calm both your body and mind.

Grounding techniques can also help you stay present and connected to the moment, reducing feelings of overwhelm. For example, focusing on your senses, describing your surroundings, or holding a comforting object can anchor you in the present and prevent your mind from spiraling into automatic responses. Cognitive restructuring is another essential strategy involving challenging and changing negative thought patterns. By recognizing when automatic negative thoughts arise and consciously replacing them with more balanced and positive thoughts, you can shift your mental framework and foster healthier emotional responses.

Build Emotional Resilience and Foster Healthier Relationship Dynamics

Building emotional resilience is crucial for long-term change and for fostering healthier relationships. Regular self-care practices are vital in maintaining your emotional and physical well-being. Engage in activities that nourish both your body and mind, such as exercise, healthy eating, and adequate sleep. Incorporating activities that bring joy and relaxation, such as hobbies, reading, or spending time in nature, is equally important.

Seeking therapeutic support can be incredibly beneficial in addressing automatic defense mechanisms. A therapist can help you explore the root causes of these responses and develop personalized strategies for change. Cognitive-behavioral therapy (CBT) or dialectical behavior therapy (DBT) are particularly effective in helping you restructure your thoughts and behaviors.

Healthy communication skills are another cornerstone of fostering positive relationship dynamics. Practice expressing your needs and feelings assertively, using "I" statements to take responsibility for your emotions. For example, instead of saying, "You make me anxious," you could say, "I feel anxious when we argue." This approach reduces blame and fosters constructive dialogue. Additionally, establishing and maintaining healthy boundaries is essential for protecting your well-being and fostering respect in relationships. Clearly communicate your boundaries and enforce them consistently. If you need time alone to recharge, communicate this need to your partner and make it a regular practice.

Building a strong support network of friends, family, or support groups is also essential. Surround yourself with people who understand and respect your journey toward healthier coping mechanisms. Participating in support groups can provide a sense of community and shared experiences, offering valuable emotional support and encouragement.

Practice Patience and Persistence
Transforming automatic defense mechanisms is a gradual process that requires patience and persistence. It's important to be gentle with yourself as you navigate this journey and to celebrate your progress along the way. Practicing self-compassion is key; treat yourself with kindness and understanding, especially when you struggle or make mistakes. Recognize that change is challenging, and it's okay to seek support when needed. Remind yourself that everyone has setbacks, and use these moments as opportunities for growth.

Consistency is crucial in creating lasting change. Commit to regularly practicing the strategies outlined above, even when it feels difficult. Over time, these new habits will become more natural and automatic. Set small, achievable goals to build momentum and track your progress. Regularly reflect on your progress and make adjustments as needed. Stay open to learning and growing, and be willing to modify your strategies to suit your evolving needs better. Celebrate your successes, no matter how small, and use them as motivation to continue your journey.

By implementing these strategies, you can effectively address automatic defense mechanisms and develop healthier ways of coping with stress and emotional challenges. This transformation will not only improve your relationships but also enhance your overall well-being and resilience.

Chapter 2 Conclusion

In Chapter 2, we explored the complex nature of automatic defense mechanisms, focusing on how these deeply ingrained responses, shaped by toxic family environments, impact our adult relationships. These defense mechanisms—whether they manifest as fight, flight, freeze, or fawn—were initially developed as survival strategies. They helped us navigate the emotional turmoil of our past, providing protection when we needed it most. However, as adults, these automatic responses often act as barriers to intimacy, trust, and genuine connection, keeping us from building the fulfilling relationships we desire.

We examined how the fight response leads to aggression and defensiveness, pushing others away during conflicts that could otherwise be resolved. The flight response manifests as avoidance or withdrawal, creating an emotional distance that leaves issues unresolved and prevents closeness. The freeze response results in emotional numbness, where you shut down completely and disengage from the relationship. Finally, the fawn response —marked by people-pleasing—causes you to prioritize your partner's needs over your own, often leading to resentment and a loss of self. In each of these cases, the brain, conditioned by past experiences, misinterprets neutral or loving interactions as threats, triggering automatic reactions that create distance instead of fostering connection.

Understanding the origins and manifestations of these defense mechanisms is crucial for anyone seeking to break free from patterns that undermine their relationships. Recognizing when your brain enters "survival mode" and how these responses play out in your interactions is the first step toward change. By identifying these automatic reactions, you can begin to interrupt the cycle and replace them with healthier coping mechanisms. This chapter introduces practical strategies like mindfulness, self-reflection, grounding techniques, and cognitive restructuring—tools that help you stay present and make conscious choices rather than reacting impulsively. These approaches are not only effective but also easy to incorporate into daily life, helping you engage with others in more authentic and emotionally available ways.

The journey to transcending these defense mechanisms requires courage, patience, and self-compassion. Change is not only possible but within reach, and it starts with the awareness that while these behaviors may have once served a protective role, they no longer serve you in the same way. With consistent effort and a commitment to personal growth, you can begin to transform these responses, breaking free from the emotional burnout, misunderstandings, and disconnection that may have characterized past relationships.

As you continue on this journey, remember to approach the process of transformation with patience. Change is gradual, and setbacks are a natural part of the process. But each step forward brings you closer to creating healthier relationship dynamics filled with deeper connections, trust, and emotional fulfillment. The insights and strategies discussed in this chapter are powerful tools that can help you reclaim your life from the shadows of your past and build relationships that truly nurture and support you.

Healing is an ongoing journey, and with every step, you move closer to the life and meaningful connections you deserve. Keep going—you have the power to create fulfilling relationships and the emotional freedom you've always hoped for.

3. Embracing Ego Death in Relationships

Building healthy intimate relationships, especially for those who have experienced toxic family dynamics, often requires a significant shift in how we see ourselves and others. Many of us have been conditioned to put others' needs before our own, leading to unhealthy dynamics where self-care is neglected. A powerful way to break this pattern is by letting go of ego-driven behaviors, such as always needing to be correct, seeking approval, trying to control situations, or struggling to admit fault. These tendencies often undermine emotional connection and create barriers to intimacy.

The ego, in this context, refers to the part of your mind that is concerned with self-importance, control, and how others perceive you. The ego is all about your perception of yourself—how you see yourself and how you believe others should see you. When someone's behavior or words don't align with the image of yourself that you hold in your mind, the ego reacts defensively, which can lead to negative emotions like anger, frustration, or resentment. This drive to protect your sense of self often results in power struggles, emotional distance, or even manipulation, preventing the emotional openness needed for a healthy relationship.

For example, think of times when you've had an argument with a partner. You may have felt an urge to defend yourself, prove your point, or control the situation. Perhaps you've focused more on winning the argument or seeking validation rather than truly listening to your partner's feelings. These ego-driven behaviors feel protective in the moment, but they often lead to emotional distance and conflict. Letting go of these impulses—learning to pause, listen, and approach your partner with empathy and vulnerability—is essential to improving your relationship dynamics.

Ego death, then, is the process of setting aside this need to protect or validate yourself constantly. It doesn't mean losing your identity; instead, it means letting go of the parts of your ego that prioritize control and validation over understanding and connection. When you embrace ego death in relationships, you shift away from ego-driven actions like needing to prove yourself or seeking to control outcomes. Instead, you focus on fostering trust, empathy, and mutual respect. By releasing the urge to dominate or defend, you make space for vulnerability and openness, the true foundations of emotional intimacy and connection.

Ultimately, embracing ego death in relationships means creating a dynamic where understanding, connection, and mutual respect take priority over control, validation, and ego-driven needs. It allows you to approach your partner with authenticity and empathy without letting the fear of losing control or being vulnerable stand in the way. Instead of losing yourself, you create space for a partnership built on mutual growth and emotional fulfillment—where both individuals are free to be themselves without the constant need for defense or approval. By letting go of the ego's grasp, you foster a relationship that thrives on genuine connection and emotional freedom.

Relationship Priorities: Self-Care and Ego Death
One of the most significant shifts you can make in your relationships is prioritizing self-care and compassion over ego-driven needs. It's easy to fall into the trap of believing that a

relationship requires self-sacrifice or putting your partner's needs ahead of your own. However, placing self-care first ensures that you bring your best self to the relationship, ultimately benefiting both you and your partner. Ego-driven desires—such as needing to be right, controlling situations, or fearing vulnerability—can undermine a relationship by creating power imbalances and emotional disconnect.

Ego death, in this context, means letting go of the desire to dominate or protect your ego within the relationship. By prioritizing self-care, you allow yourself to release the need for control and instead embrace vulnerability, trust, and openness. This shift enables both you and your partner to grow together without the tension that arises from ego-driven actions. When you focus on nurturing your well-being first, the relationship naturally becomes stronger, as both partners feel supported, respected, and seen for who they truly are.

Ultimately, embracing ego death in relationships creates a dynamic where mutual respect and connection are prioritized over control and validation. By ensuring self-care comes first, you build a foundation for a relationship that is balanced, sustainable, and fulfilling. Rather than losing yourself in the needs of the relationship, you maintain your sense of identity while fostering a partnership rooted in mutual growth, empathy, and emotional well-being.

Understanding the Concept of Ego Death

The concept of "ego death" is explored in various psychological and philosophical traditions, often referring to a profound shift in one's sense of self or identity. In psychology, this idea is sometimes discussed in terms of self-transcendence, where an individual moves beyond the limited perspective of the ego—the part of the mind tied to self-identity, personal desires, and attachment to specific outcomes. Transcending ego-driven behaviors in relationships is essential because it enables individuals to connect more authentically and meaningfully, fostering relationships based on mutual respect, understanding, and emotional depth.

Examples of Ego-Driven Behaviors

Here are some examples of ego-driven behaviors:

Need for Control

In relationships, the ego often drives a desire to control situations, outcomes, or even the other person. For example, insisting on making all decisions or needing to know every detail of your partner's day can be ego-driven behaviors. This need for control stems from a fear of vulnerability and uncertainty, where the ego equates control with safety and security. However, this can lead to tension and resentment, as it undermines your partner's autonomy and the natural flow of the relationship.

Seeking Validation

Another common ego-driven behavior is the constant need for validation from your partner. This might manifest as frequently asking for reassurance, needing compliments, or relying on your partner to boost your self-esteem. For instance, if you feel insecure about your appearance or achievements, you might seek continuous praise to feel worthy. While occasional validation is normal, relying on it excessively can strain the relationship, as it places undue pressure on your partner to constantly affirm your value.

Fear of Criticism or Rejection

The ego is sensitive to criticism and often reacts defensively when it perceives a threat to self-esteem. In a relationship, this might look like becoming overly defensive during disagreements, refusing to accept constructive feedback, or avoiding difficult conversations altogether. For example, if your partner points out a behavior that bothers them, you might respond by shutting down or lashing out instead of listening and engaging in a constructive dialogue. This defensiveness can prevent growth and understanding within the relationship.

Jealousy and Possessiveness

Jealousy often stems from the ego's fear of losing something it values, like attention or a sense of control. In relationships, this can manifest as possessiveness, where you may feel threatened by your partner's interactions with others, even if they are harmless. For example, if your partner spends time with friends or colleagues, you might feel insecure and demand constant updates or reassurance. The ego drives this behavior because it focuses on protecting the self from perceived threats rather than trusting in the stability and mutual respect of the relationship.

Reluctance to Apologize

The ego can make it difficult to admit when you're wrong or to apologize sincerely. In relationships, this might manifest as stubbornness, where you hold onto your position even when it's clear that you've made a mistake. For example, if you've had an argument with your partner and realize you were in the wrong, the ego might resist acknowledging this, fearing that admitting fault will diminish your self-worth. This reluctance to apologize can prevent resolution and healing in the relationship.

Resentment and Holding Grudges

Resentment is often born from the ego's sense of injustice or feeling undervalued. When someone feels wronged or hurt in a relationship, rather than addressing the issue openly, they may allow those negative feelings to fester. This is an ego-driven response because it centers on self-protection and a desire to hold onto past grievances instead of seeking resolution or understanding. Resentment often builds up over time, creating emotional distance and deepening the divide in the relationship.

In toxic relationships, resentment can become a recurring pattern. Instead of expressing concerns or boundaries in a healthy way, individuals may bottle up their frustrations, allowing them to surface in passive-aggressive behavior or emotional withdrawal. The ego feeds off these negative emotions, focusing on the perceived unfairness or mistreatment, which prevents the person from moving forward or healing. This pattern can make it nearly impossible to foster a healthy connection, as resentment poisons the emotional environment between partners.

Breaking free from resentment requires letting go of the ego's grip on past wrongs. It involves learning to communicate openly and honestly about your feelings and recognizing that holding onto anger only keeps you stuck in a cycle of bitterness. By practicing empathy and understanding, you can release the need to hold onto past grievances and instead focus on building a relationship rooted in mutual respect and emotional healing.

Why Transcending Ego-Driven Behaviors Matters
Transcending these ego-driven behaviors is essential for building a healthy, fulfilling relationship. When you move beyond the ego's demands for control, validation, and self-protection, you open yourself up to a more genuine connection with your partner. This shift allows you to engage with them from a place of mutual respect, trust, and empathy rather than from fear or insecurity. By letting go of the ego's grip, you create space for a deeper, more authentic relationship where both partners can grow and thrive together.

Related Concepts in Psychology and Literature
Here are some related concepts found in psychology and literature:
- **Ego Dissolution:** In psychological literature, particularly in studies related to mindfulness, meditation, and psychedelics, "ego dissolution" is a term used to describe the temporary experience of losing the boundaries of the ego. During this state, individuals may feel a deep sense of interconnectedness with others or the universe, free from the usual constraints of personal identity.

- **Self-Transcendence:** Abraham Maslow, known for his hierarchy of needs, spoke of self-transcendence as a stage where individuals go beyond self-actualization. This stage involves transcending the ego and experiencing a connection to something greater, whether that's other people, nature, or a higher purpose.
- **Anatta (No-Self):** In Buddhist philosophy, the concept of "anatta" or "no-self" is central. It suggests that the self is an illusion and clinging to the ego is a source of suffering. The path to enlightenment involves recognizing and overcoming this attachment to the self, leading to greater peace and compassion.
- **Ego Death in Mysticism and Spirituality:** In various mystical and spiritual traditions, "ego death" refers to a profound experience where the individual feels as though their ego, or sense of separate self, has dissolved. This can lead to a heightened state of awareness, unity with the universe, or a deep sense of inner peace.
- **Depersonalization and Derealization:** In some psychological conditions, such as depersonalization or derealization, individuals might feel detached from their sense of self or reality, which can resemble aspects of ego death. However, unlike the spiritually or therapeutically sought-after ego dissolution, these experiences can be distressing and are considered symptoms of certain mental health conditions.

Applying "Death to the Ego" in Relationships

In the context of relationships, the idea of "death to the ego" can be about letting go of the need to control outcomes, seek validation, or protect one's self-image. It involves approaching interactions with others from a place of humility, openness, and compassion rather than from the ego-driven desires for recognition or superiority. This concept encourages individuals to prioritize self-care, self-compassion, and the well-being of the relationship over the ego's demands, leading to healthier, more fulfilling connections.

By embracing this idea, you can move toward a more balanced and authentic way of being, where the ego's influence is diminished, and you are free to engage in relationships and life with greater peace and presence.

Embracing Death to Ego: The Path to Healthy Relationships

By embracing the concept of ego death, you dismantle the barriers that often hinder genuine connection and emotional intimacy. When the ego is set aside, the need to control outcomes, win arguments, or protect your image at the expense of the relationship fades away. Instead, decisions are made from a place of compassion, understanding, and mutual respect. This shift fosters more authentic communication, deeper understanding, and a stronger bond between partners.

Ego death in relationships leads to a more balanced dynamic where both individuals feel valued and respected. It reduces conflicts driven by insecurity or the need to assert dominance, replacing them with interactions rooted in empathy and cooperation. In this environment, both partners are free to grow, both as individuals and within the relationship, leading to healthier, more fulfilling connections.

Incorporating these priorities into your relationship—putting self-care first and the relationship second while embracing ego death—creates a powerful framework for lasting partnership and mutual growth. By focusing on these principles, you can navigate your relationship with confidence, knowing that you are building it on a foundation of strength, respect, and genuine connection.

Ego and Its Role in Relationships

Understanding the role of ego in relationships is key to navigating the complex dynamics that often arise, especially in the context of healing from a toxic family background. The ego can be thought of as that part of ourselves that craves validation, control, and the need to be right. In relationships, this can manifest as defensiveness, a desire to dominate, or an inability to compromise. The ego, when unchecked, often prioritizes self-preservation over mutual understanding and growth.

In relationships shaped by toxic family dynamics, the ego often develops as a protective mechanism. For example, in an environment where acceptance and approval were conditional, the ego may have become hyper-vigilant, constantly guarding against perceived threats. However, in adult relationships, this same ego-driven behavior can become a barrier to genuine connection and emotional closeness.

Healing from Toxic Family Dynamics Through Death to Ego
Growing up in a toxic family environment often involves navigating complex dynamics where control, manipulation, and power struggles are prevalent. In such settings, the ego develops as a defense mechanism—a way to survive in an environment where self-worth is constantly challenged. As a result, in adult relationships, this ego-driven approach can continue, leading to a fear of vulnerability, difficulty letting go of control, and an overemphasis on outcomes.

In the context of healing from toxic family influences, putting the ego to death means consciously choosing to step back from these ingrained patterns. It involves recognizing when your decisions are being driven by fear, insecurity, or the need to protect your image and, instead, choosing a path of humility, openness, and mutual respect. This shift allows you to approach relationships from a place of wholeness and security rather than from a place of neediness or fear.

Detaching from Outcomes and

the Need for Validation

Detaching from Outcomes and the Need for Validation

Growing up in a toxic family environment often instills a deep-seated need for validation and a strong attachment to specific outcomes. In such settings, approval and acceptance may have been conditional, leading you to equate success, external recognition, and meeting others' expectations with your personal worth. This conditioning often carries over into adult relationships, where attachment to outcomes and a constant need for validation can create unnecessary stress, anxiety, and a fragile sense of self-worth. Overcoming these patterns is essential for healing and building healthier, more genuine connections.

Understanding Ego-Driven Attachments

The ego thrives on control and recognition. When you attach your sense of self to the success of a relationship, a career milestone, or a personal goal, you're essentially placing your worth in the hands of external circumstances. The ego tells you that if things go well, you're worthy and valuable; if they don't, you're less so. This creates a cycle of anxiety, as you're constantly striving to achieve or maintain outcomes that you believe define your identity.

It's crucial to recognize that the need for validation is rooted in the ego's desire to be seen, acknowledged, and praised. Whether it's approval from a partner, recognition at work, or likes on social media, the ego craves external affirmation to reinforce a positive self-image. This recognition is the first step to understanding its power over you. However, when your sense of worth is tied to how others perceive you, it becomes fragile and dependent on factors beyond your control. This can lead to a constant need for reassurance, leaving you feeling unfulfilled and insecure when that validation is absent.

Letting Go of Control and Specific Outcomes

Letting go of control and specific outcomes is a crucial part of healing toxic relationships. It means accepting that you cannot dictate every aspect of your life or relationships and recognizing that real connection and personal growth come from allowing both yourself and others to grow and thrive independently. When you release the need to control outcomes, you make decisions from a place of respect and self-awareness rather than trying to protect the ego. This approach is not about abandoning your goals or values but about embracing flexibility and resilience in the face of life's uncertainties, empowering you to navigate challenges with greater confidence and clarity.

The Pitfalls of Ego-Driven Behaviors

Attachment to outcomes and the need for validation can create several pitfalls in relationships and personal growth. When you're overly attached to a specific outcome, any deviation from your expectations can cause emotional distress. This often leads to frustration, disappointment, and even resentment—toward both yourself and others. In relationships, this can manifest as pressure on your partner to meet certain standards or expectations, which strains the connection.

The need for validation can also foster a perpetual state of insecurity, as your self-worth becomes contingent on others' opinions. This constant need for approval can lead to persistent anxiety, leaving you wondering if you're doing enough or if others approve of you. Such anxiety hinders your ability to be authentic and present in your relationships.

Additionally, when the ego is fixated on specific outcomes, it can limit your ability to embrace new experiences and learn from them. Growth often requires letting go of preconceived notions and being open to unexpected paths. The ego's attachment to a single outcome can prevent you from recognizing opportunities for growth in failure or change.

Cultivating Detachment and Self-Compassion

Detaching from outcomes and the need for validation doesn't mean you stop caring about your goals or relationships. Instead, it involves shifting your focus from external results and approval to internal values and self-worth. The process begins with practicing self-awareness. Start by recognizing when your ego is driving your thoughts and actions. Ask yourself if you are overly concerned with how others perceive you or if you're fixated on a particular outcome. This awareness is the first step to change.

Next, embrace the present moment. Rather than focusing on future outcomes, turn your attention to the here and now. Engage fully in whatever you're doing—whether it's working on a project, spending time with someone important, or pursuing a goal. By staying present, you'll appreciate the journey instead of obsessing over the destination.

It's also important to develop internal validation. Cultivate a sense of self-worth that isn't reliant on external approval. Remind yourself that your value comes from who you are, not from what you achieve or how others view you. Practice self-compassion regularly and affirm your inherent worth.

Another key aspect is letting go of control. Accept that not everything is within your control. Outcomes are influenced by various factors, some of which are beyond your reach. By releasing the need to control every aspect of your life, you reduce stress and open yourself to new possibilities.

Finally, reframe failure and change. Instead of seeing them as threats to your ego, view them as opportunities for growth. Each experience, whether it meets your expectations or not, offers valuable lessons that contribute to your personal development.

Detaching from outcomes and the need for validation allows you to live more authentically and freely. By reducing the influence of the ego, you create space for deeper connections, greater resilience, and a more fulfilling life. In your relationships, this detachment fosters a healthier dynamic, where connection is based on mutual respect and understanding rather than on meeting expectations or seeking approval. Ultimately, adopting this mindset leads to a more balanced, peaceful, and empowered way of being.

Practical Steps for Embracing Ego Death in Relationships

Embracing ego death in relationships is a transformative process that goes beyond merely understanding the concept; it requires deliberate, ongoing action. The journey toward healthier, more fulfilling connections begins with the conscious decision to let go of ego-driven behaviors in favor of empathy, collaboration, and mutual growth. By integrating practical strategies into your daily life, you can create a relationship dynamic that prioritizes the well-being of both individuals and thrives on respect, understanding, and authentic connection.

Mindfulness and Self-Reflection

Incorporating mindfulness and regular self-reflection into your daily routine can help you recognize when your ego is influencing your behavior. Ask yourself: "Am I making this decision out of fear or a need to protect my ego, or am I prioritizing self-care and the health of the relationship?" This self-awareness is the first step toward change, allowing you to make more conscious, loving choices.

Open and Honest Communication

Creating a space for open and honest communication with your partner is vital. When both partners can express their needs, fears, and desires without judgment or ego interference, it fosters a deeper connection and mutual understanding. This practice helps dismantle the barriers that the ego often erects.

Embrace Vulnerability

Rather than seeing vulnerability as a weakness, view it as a strength—an opportunity to connect with your partner on a deeper level. For example, instead of insisting on being right in a disagreement, choose to listen and understand your partner's perspective. Embracing vulnerability in this way fosters deeper connection and trust.

Let Go of the Need to Be Right
In situations where you might typically insist on being right or having the last word, consciously choose to prioritize the health of the relationship over the need to win. This practice encourages compromise and collaboration, strengthening your bond with your partner.

Prioritize the Relationship Over Self-Image
There may be times when protecting your self-image could lead to defensiveness or withdrawal. Instead, focus on the relationship's well-being. This might mean apologizing when you're wrong, admitting when you're unsure, or being open about your insecurities. Such honesty can bring you closer together and reduce unnecessary conflicts.

Commit to Self-Care
Prioritizing your own well-being is the foundation for a healthy relationship. When you take care of yourself, you are less likely to rely on your partner to meet all your emotional needs. This reduces the burden on the relationship and allows both partners to thrive individually and together.

Foster Mutual Growth
Encourage a dynamic where both partners can grow and evolve. Support each other's goals and aspirations, and celebrate one another's achievements. By focusing on mutual growth rather than competing or comparing, you create a relationship environment where both individuals feel valued and respected.

By integrating these practical steps into your daily life, you can create a relationship dynamic that is rooted in respect, mutual growth, and understanding. Letting go of ego in relationships is an ongoing process, but with commitment and practice, it leads to a more fulfilling and resilient partnership.

Chapter 3 Conclusion

In this chapter, we explored the transformative power of embracing ego death as a fundamental principle for building healthier, more resilient relationships. Ego death, which involves letting go of the need for control, validation, and constant self-protection, allows you to create a relationship built on trust, empathy, and mutual respect. This shift in focus—from protecting yourself to fostering connection—paves the way for deeper intimacy and emotional fulfillment.

When you let go of ego-driven behaviors like needing to win arguments, control situations, or protect your self-image, you create space for genuine communication and understanding. Rather than approaching your relationship with defensiveness or fear, you can engage with openness and vulnerability, which strengthens the bond between you and your partner. This shift helps you avoid the common pitfalls of ego-driven relationships —power struggles, emotional distance, and manipulation—and instead fosters an environment where both partners can thrive together.

The process of embracing ego death is not about losing yourself but about releasing the parts of your ego that hinder connection. By stepping away from the urge to defend or validate your sense of self constantly, you allow your relationship to grow from a place of authenticity. This allows for a dynamic where both partners are free to be themselves without the need for control or domination, leading to a stronger, more fulfilling partnership.

Healing from a toxic family background often involves unlearning the ego-driven behaviors that once served as survival mechanisms. Reclaiming your power in relationships means consciously choosing to set aside these automatic defenses and instead focus on trust, emotional availability, and mutual respect. By embracing ego death, you take control of your role in creating the loving, supportive relationships you deserve—ones that are rooted in mutual growth and respect rather than fear or self-preservation.

As you move forward on this journey, remember that letting go of ego is a practice that requires patience and daily mindfulness. It involves staying aware of your reactions, your motivations, and your impulses to control or seek validation. But with each step toward ego death, you open yourself up to deeper intimacy, stronger connections, and the opportunity for both you and your partner to flourish together in harmony. Through this ongoing process, you create relationships that are not only strong but deeply nourishing and sustainable.

4. Understanding Dependency and Codependency

rowing up in a toxic family environment often results in deep-seated patterns of unhealthy dependency and codependency. These patterns, formed in childhood, can profoundly impact adult relationships, creating dynamics that are challenging to navigate and detrimental to both partners' well-being. Understanding and addressing these issues is crucial for building healthier, more fulfilling relationships.

Unhealthy Dependency and Codependency

Toxic family backgrounds frequently contribute to the development of unhealthy dependency and codependency. In such environments, children may learn to rely excessively on others for validation, security, and a sense of self-worth. This dependency can stem from inconsistent support, emotional manipulation, or neglect. As these children grow into adults, they may carry these patterns into their relationships, seeking constant reassurance and validation from their partners, often at the expense of their own independence and emotional health.

Codependency, on the other hand, is a pattern where individuals place the needs and desires of others above their own, often to the point of self-neglect. In toxic families, codependent behaviors develop as coping mechanisms, where individuals learn to prioritize the emotional states of others to maintain stability and avoid conflict. These behaviors persist in adult relationships, leading to unbalanced dynamics where one partner becomes overly reliant on the other for emotional fulfillment.

"I'm Not Good Enough"

At the heart of both dependency and codependency lies a powerful core belief: "I'm not good enough." This negative self-perception drives much of the behavior associated with these dynamics in relationships. Dependent individuals often struggle with making decisions independently because they inherently doubt their judgment and capabilities. They may find themselves constantly seeking their partner's input and approval, not because they lack the ability to decide for themselves but because they lack the confidence to trust their own decisions.

This belief creates a cycle of reliance. Dependent individuals may feel that they need their partner to complete them, validate their worth, and reassure them of their place in the world. Without their partner's constant affirmation, they may feel incomplete, insecure, and unworthy.

In codependency, the belief of I'm not good enough" drives the caretaker's behavior. They derive their sense of self-worth from taking care of others, often neglecting their own needs in the process. They may believe that by keeping others happy or taking on the role of the "fixer," they can maintain stability in relationships and avoid rejection or abandonment. This dynamic reinforces their self-perception as only valuable when they are needed by others, further entrenching the belief that they aren't inherently worthy on their own.

Addressing this negative core belief is essential for breaking the cycles of dependency and codependency. Recognizing the belief and understanding how it influences behavior can be the first step toward developing a healthier, more balanced sense of self.

Internalized Beliefs and Self-Worth

The messages conveyed by toxic family dynamics can severely impact an individual's self-worth. Children raised in such environments often internalize beliefs that they are not good enough, that their needs are less important, and that they must constantly prove their value to be accepted. These deeply ingrained beliefs shape their self-concept and how they engage with others, often leading to unhealthy relationship patterns and difficulty asserting their own needs.

In adult relationships, these internalized beliefs manifest as dependency and codependency. Dependent individuals may struggle with low self-esteem and constantly seek external validation to feel secure. Codependent individuals may derive their self-worth from being needed and taking care of others, often at the expense of their own well-being.

Patterns of Dependency and Codependency
An excessive need for reassurance, approval, and support from a partner characterizes unhealthy dependency in relationships. Dependent individuals may have difficulty making decisions independently and constantly seek their partner's input and validation. They may fear being alone and feel incomplete without their partner's presence.

Codependency takes this a step further, where individuals not only rely on their partners but also feel responsible for their emotions and actions. Codependent individuals may go to great lengths to keep their partner happy, even if it means sacrificing their own needs and desires. They might engage in enabling behaviors, where they try to fix or rescue their partner from problems, believing that their worth is tied to their partner's well-being.

Breaking the Cycle
Understanding how toxic family dynamics contribute to unhealthy dependency and codependency is the first step toward breaking the cycle. It requires recognizing these patterns and their

origins, challenging internalized beliefs, and developing healthier ways of relating to others. This process involves building self-esteem, setting boundaries, and learning to prioritize one's own needs without feeling guilty or unworthy.

Strategies for Healthy Dependency

Breaking free from unhealthy dependency and codependency requires intentional effort, self-awareness, and the development of healthy habits. Cultivating a healthier form of dependency involves recognizing patterns, fostering independence, and building emotional resilience. Below are essential strategies that can help you transform your relationships:

Develop Self-Awareness and Self-Reflection

The first step toward breaking free from unhealthy dependency is recognizing the patterns in your relationships. Take time to reflect on how often you seek validation or reassurance from your partner and what situations trigger these behaviors. Self-awareness is critical because it allows you to identify the root causes of dependency, such as past trauma or a lack of self-confidence. Keeping a journal or engaging in mindfulness practices can help you become more aware of your thoughts and behaviors, allowing you to gain insight into your emotional needs. With this awareness, you can begin the journey of change.

Build Self-Confidence and Self-Esteem

Strengthening your self-esteem is essential for reducing dependency on others. Low self-esteem often fuels the need for external validation, leading you to rely on your partner to feel good about yourself. To break this cycle, engage in activities that challenge you and boost your confidence. Setting small, achievable goals can help you experience personal success and build a sense of competence and self-worth. Surround yourself with positive influences—people who encourage your growth and affirm your abilities. Over time, you will begin to develop the confidence to make decisions and stand on your own without constantly seeking approval from others.

Foster Emotional Independence

Emotional independence is about learning to regulate your emotions and manage stress without relying on others to calm or reassure you. Mindfulness practices, such as meditation, deep breathing exercises, or journaling, are effective ways to process difficult emotions on your own. Emotional independence doesn't mean cutting yourself off from others, but it allows you to handle stress, disappointment, and uncertainty in a healthy way without becoming overly reliant on your partner. As you cultivate emotional resilience, you'll find it easier to face challenges independently, strengthening your relationship by removing the pressure on your partner to meet all of your emotional needs.

Set Healthy Boundaries

Establishing and maintaining boundaries is crucial for preventing enmeshment and promoting mutual respect in a relationship. Healthy boundaries allow both partners to have space for their individuality while maintaining connection. Be clear and honest with your partner about your personal limits—whether it's emotional, physical, or psychological—and ensure that both of you respect each other's boundaries. Boundaries not only protect your well-being but also promote a sense of security and trust within the relationship. Learning to say "no" when necessary and standing firm in your boundaries will prevent the unhealthy dynamics that lead to dependency and codependency.

Pursue Personal Interests and Hobbies

Maintaining your individuality is key to fostering healthy dependency. Engaging in hobbies, interests, and activities that bring you joy and fulfillment allows you to maintain a sense of self apart from your relationship. Personal interests help you stay connected to your own identity and provide a sense of accomplishment outside of your partnership. Whether it's pursuing a creative hobby, fitness routine, or professional goal, having time to yourself enriches your life and reinforces your emotional independence. Prioritizing these interests also shows that you value yourself, which ultimately strengthens the relationship.

Communicate Openly and Honestly

Effective communication is foundational to any healthy relationship, particularly in overcoming dependency and codependency. Openly express your needs, concerns, and emotions with your partner in a way that encourages mutual understanding and respect. When communication is clear and honest, it fosters trust and reduces the likelihood of misunderstandings or unmet expectations. Practice active listening as well, giving your partner the space to share their thoughts without judgment. This two-way exchange builds a solid foundation of support, ensuring that both partners feel heard and valued, rather than one person being overly dependent on the other for validation.

Seek Professional Support

Sometimes, the patterns of dependency and codependency are deeply ingrained, requiring additional help to overcome. Therapy is a valuable resource for those struggling with these issues. A therapist can guide you in identifying the unhealthy dynamics in your relationship and help you develop the skills needed to foster a more balanced and fulfilling partnership. Therapy can also provide a safe space for processing emotions and breaking free from patterns that no longer serve you. By working with a professional, you gain valuable tools to improve your emotional health and create healthier, more sustainable relationships.

Addressing the root causes of dependency and codependency takes effort, but the rewards are profound. By developing self-awareness, building self-confidence, fostering emotional independence, and setting boundaries, you can cultivate healthier relationships that allow for both personal growth and mutual support. As you implement these strategies, you will find a greater balance in your connections—one where both you and your partner can thrive individually and together. With time and commitment, the journey toward healthy dependency can lead to relationships that are both fulfilling and resilient.

Chapter 4 Conclusion

In this chapter, we explore the transformative potential of understanding how toxic family environments often lead to unhealthy patterns of dependency and codependency. These patterns, deeply rooted in childhood experiences, can profoundly impact adult relationships. However, by understanding these dynamics, you can take the first step towards transforming your relationships and achieving healthier, more fulfilling connections.

At the heart of dependency and codependency lies a powerful belief: "I'm not good enough." This belief drives behaviors of seeking constant validation or caretaking, often at the expense of individuality and personal growth. However, recognizing this belief and its influence on your interactions can empower you to break free from cycles of reliance and self-doubt.

We also examined the ways toxic family dynamics shape dependency and codependency through emotional inconsistency, manipulation, and neglect. These early experiences teach individuals to rely excessively on others for validation and support. However, breaking the cycle is possible with self-awareness and the implementation of healthy strategies.

Through practical steps like building self-confidence, fostering emotional independence, and setting boundaries, you can cultivate a healthier relationship dynamic. Engaging in personal interests, improving communication, and seeking professional support are also key to developing healthier relationships where both partners thrive.

In summary, overcoming unhealthy dependency and codependency is a journey that requires commitment and intentional effort. By addressing the root causes of these behaviors, you can foster relationships where personal growth and mutual support coexist, allowing you to form deep connections without sacrificing your sense of self.

5. The Need for Personal Space in Intimate Relationships

Many people often confuse the concepts of dependency or codependency with the time spent apart from a partner, assuming that personal space means physically distancing oneself. However, the real issue lies more in the mindset of maintaining your authentic self within the relationship rather than how much time you spend together. Dependency and codependency are rooted in losing sight of your individual identity, relying on your partner to meet all your emotional needs, or trying to control their behaviors to feel secure. Personal space, on the other hand, is not about separation or detachment but about creating room to grow as an individual while still nurturing the relationship.

Growing up in a toxic family environment can leave lasting scars that shape how you relate to others, often leading to patterns of insecurity, dependency, or fear of abandonment. In families where emotional needs were unmet or relationships were built on control and manipulation, the idea of personal space might feel foreign or even threatening. Many people who come from these backgrounds may find it difficult to establish healthy boundaries in their adult relationships, either clinging too tightly to their partner or withdrawing when conflict arises.

These early experiences can create a constant need for validation or reassurance from others, which makes it hard to feel secure when you or your partner needs time alone. This can lead to emotional burnout, tension, and misunderstandings, as one partner may feel suffocated while the other feels neglected. Without space, relationships can become strained because there's no room for personal growth, reflection, or self-care—key elements of maintaining emotional health.

The need for personal space in intimate relationships is not a sign of weakness or disconnection; rather, it's a necessary part of a healthy, balanced relationship. Time apart allows you to recharge, process your emotions, and tend to your own needs without losing sight of your partner. For those who grew up in chaotic or controlling family environments, learning to respect personal space can feel uncomfortable at first, but it's essential for building stronger, healthier relationships based on mutual trust and respect.

In this chapter, we will explore the importance of creating both physical and emotional space within a relationship. By establishing clear boundaries and openly communicating your needs, you foster an environment where both partners can thrive as individuals while maintaining a strong emotional connection. Personal space is not about withdrawing from your partner but about creating room for each person to grow, reflect, and nurture their well-being—ultimately leading to a more fulfilling and sustainable relationship.

You don't have to leave your partner's presence to maintain personal space physically. It could mean engaging in different activities, like reading or pursuing a hobby, while still being in the same room or simply agreeing on quiet time where each person can focus inward. Creating mental and emotional space while staying physically close helps maintain balance and independence, allowing both partners to feel secure without needing constant interaction. These small moments of personal space, even while sharing physical proximity, can deepen your connection and enhance your individual well-being.

Ultimately, the most important aspect of maintaining personal space in any intimate relationship is staying true to your authentic self. By nurturing your own identity, needs, and emotional well-being, you create a stronger foundation for your relationship. When both partners are able to bring their full, genuine selves into the relationship, it fosters mutual growth, deeper intimacy, and a more balanced, respectful partnership. Remember, honoring your own individuality not only benefits you but also strengthens the bond you share with your partner, allowing the relationship to flourish.

Staying True to Your Authentic Self in Relationships

Maintaining personal space in intimate relationships is not just about physical distance—it's about preserving your authentic self, even in the closest connections. When you remain connected to your own identity, needs, and emotional well-being, you lay the foundation for a stronger, healthier relationship. For many who come from toxic family backgrounds, it's easy to lose sight of your individual self in relationships. Dependency or fear of abandonment can cause you to rely too heavily on your partner, making it difficult to maintain your sense of identity. The most important aspect of personal space, therefore, is staying true to who you are, even in moments of closeness.

Growing up in a toxic family environment, I often resolved my feelings of pain, anger, fear, and resentment by physically distancing myself from my family members. It was my way of protecting myself—whenever the tension became unbearable, I would retreat to find some sense of peace. This survival mechanism helped me in my childhood, but as I grew older, I realized that I was carrying this habit into my adult relationships. Whenever things became emotionally intense with a partner, my first instinct was to withdraw, believing that space was the only way I could feel safe.

However, this approach led to emotional distance and misunderstandings, often leaving me disconnected from the people I cared about. I soon realized that I wasn't truly engaging with those around me, nor was I expressing my authentic self. I was simply avoiding discomfort. To build healthier relationships, I had to learn how to stay present and grounded even during challenging moments without relying on emotional withdrawal as my default coping mechanism.

Mindfulness became a crucial tool in this transformation. Instead of distancing myself, I learned to use mindfulness practices to ground myself in the present moment. These practices helped me recognize when I was reacting to old emotional triggers from my past rather than the reality of my current relationship. By tuning into my emotional responses, I could stay present with my partner without shutting down or retreating. I discovered that personal space wasn't about escaping but about creating mental and emotional room for myself, even while staying physically close.

Practical Strategies for Creating Personal Space While Staying Connected
Here are some practical strategies for maintaining personal space while staying connected in your intimate relationships. These approaches help you process emotions, find inner calm, and nurture your authentic self, all while remaining present with your partner. Each of these techniques encourages mindfulness, balance, and emotional resilience, allowing you to maintain closeness without feeling overwhelmed or losing your sense of individuality.

Engaging in Quiet Activities
You don't always need to leave the room to find personal space. Engaging in calming, quiet activities such as reading, journaling, knitting, or meditating can help you create emotional space while still being in your partner's presence. This allows you to reflect

and recharge without withdrawing completely, offering a mental retreat while staying physically close.

Breathing Exercises and Mindfulness

Practicing deep breathing, body scans, or short mindfulness exercises when emotions run high can help you center yourself. These techniques create an internal sense of space, helping you manage emotional reactions while remaining fully present with your partner. A few moments of mindful breathing can help diffuse tension and give you the clarity to respond with calmness and empathy.

Practicing Shared Silence

Agreeing with your partner to have moments of silence while sitting together can be a powerful way to create emotional space. This could mean sitting quietly with each other, perhaps reading or reflecting, without the need for conversation. Shared silence allows both partners to focus inward without feeling the need to fill the space with words, fostering a deeper connection through mutual respect for each other's inner world.

Gentle Physical Touch

Sometimes, simple acts of affection—like holding hands, a light touch, or resting your head on your partner's shoulder—can help create emotional space without saying a word. This kind of connection offers reassurance while allowing both partners to find stillness and emotional balance, reinforcing that space doesn't have to mean distance.

Creating Physical Space Within the Same Room

It's okay to take up separate corners of the same space. For example, you might sit on different sides of the room while working on individual activities. This allows each person to maintain their personal space while still sharing physical proximity, respecting the need for individual mental space while staying connected.

Using Affirmations or Self-Reflection

Practicing self-compassion through positive affirmations or silent self-reflection can help you process difficult emotions. You can do this quietly while in your partner's presence, focusing on grounding yourself emotionally and reinforcing your sense of self, all while maintaining closeness.

Listening to Calming Music or Ambient Sounds

Creating a peaceful environment through calming music or ambient sounds can provide a shared yet soothing space where both partners can relax and decompress without needing to interact directly. Music can offer emotional comfort, helping you both to reflect, breathe, and find inner calm while staying present together.

Practicing Eye Contact or Non-Verbal Communication

Sometimes, staying connected without words can offer a sense of personal space and emotional clarity. Practicing mindful eye contact or non-verbal communication like a smile, a nod, or a gentle touch allows you to remain connected to your partner while giving both of you the space to process emotions without the pressure of verbal conversation.

Being Together While Doing Separate Activities on Your Phones

You and your partner can be in each other's presence while each of you is on your own phone or device, engaging in separate activities. Some believe that phones should be put away when you're together, but in reality, using devices separately can provide a way to exist in a shared environment while still enjoying personal activities. From a psychological standpoint, this allows you to pursue independent activities while benefiting from the proximity and emotional connection that comes from simply being near each other. It respects each partner's need for mental space while reinforcing a sense of togetherness without the need for constant interaction. It's another way to find balance between closeness and individuality.

By incorporating these strategies into your daily life, you can create personal space without needing physical distance from your partner. These practices help ensure you nurture both your individual well-being and the emotional connection you share, allowing your relationship to flourish in a way that honors both partners' needs.

From an attachment theory perspective, shared screen time while being in each other's presence can foster a sense of security and emotional connection, even when partners are not directly engaging. In secure attachment styles, individuals feel comfortable with both closeness and independence. This means they can enjoy separate activities without feeling disconnected or anxious about their partner's absence. Shared screen time allows couples to maintain physical proximity, which strengthens the emotional bond while still honoring their individual need for mental space and autonomy. By being near each other without the constant pressure to interact, both partners are reminded of the secure base their relationship provides, helping them feel emotionally safe.

This balance of independence and closeness is particularly beneficial for avoiding anxious or avoidant attachment behaviors. For those with anxious attachment styles, shared screen time can offer reassurance that their partner is present without the need for continuous engagement. For avoidantly attached individuals, it can provide the necessary personal space without making them feel like they are abandoning the relationship. Ultimately, this practice reinforces the idea that intimacy doesn't always require direct interaction and that emotional safety and connection can be felt even during moments of independence.

Ultimately, maintaining personal space is about finding ways to honor who you are and what you need, even within close relationships. When both individuals are able to respect and create space for themselves, the relationship becomes stronger, more balanced, and far more sustainable. Staying true to your authentic self is not just a gift to yourself—it's a crucial element in building a relationship that fosters mutual growth, respect, and deep emotional connection.

Finding your authentic self, even in the midst of your intimate relationships, is the key to creating the healthy space you need to thrive. When you remain grounded in who you are, you are better equipped to manage any negative emotions that arise without relying too heavily on your partner or withdrawing completely. Over-reliance on your partner to fulfill all your emotional needs creates dependency, while running away from conflict or discomfort distances you from the potential for genuine connection. Neither of these approaches offers the balance or fulfillment that healthy relationships need.

Being your authentic self and finding personal space, even while in the presence of others, is a practice of self-awareness and emotional resilience. It allows you to navigate the complexities of your emotions without losing yourself or sacrificing the relationship. By honoring your individuality and maintaining mental and emotional space, you cultivate a partnership where both you and your partner can grow, support each other, and face challenges with mutual respect and understanding. This balance is not only the foundation for a thriving relationship but also the cornerstone of your personal well-being and emotional freedom.

Over-Reliance on Constant Companionship

A common issue for individuals raised in toxic family environments is an over-reliance on constant companionship. This dependency stems from a fear of independence and a hypersensitivity to invalidation. In a toxic family, emotional needs are often neglected, and validation is sporadic or conditional. As a result, individuals may develop an intense need for constant companionship to feel secure and validated.

This over-reliance can manifest in various ways. You might find yourself constantly seeking reassurance from your partner, feeling anxious when alone, or needing to be in constant communication with others. This dependency can strain relationships, placing an undue burden on your partner to meet all your emotional needs. It can also lead to feelings of suffocation and resentment on both sides, ultimately weakening the relationship.

The Necessity of Personal Space and Time Apart

Personal space and time apart are essential components of a healthy relationship. They allow individuals to recharge, reflect, and pursue their interests and personal growth. Time apart does not mean emotional distance; instead, it provides the space needed to maintain a sense of self and prevent enmeshment, where individual identities become blurred.

Having personal space helps you maintain your individuality and fosters a sense of self-worth that is not solely dependent on your relationship. It also encourages healthy interdependence, where both partners support each other while maintaining their independence. This balance is crucial for a thriving relationship, as it ensures that both partners are contributing to the relationship from a place of wholeness and self-assuredness.

Understanding the necessity of personal space involves recognizing the signs of when you or your partner need time apart. These signs can include feeling overwhelmed, irritable, or overly dependent on each other for emotional validation. Respecting these needs for space can strengthen the relationship by preventing burnout and promoting a healthy dynamic of support and individuality.

Strategies for Healthy Independence

Balancing time together with personal independence is essential for maintaining a healthy relationship. This requires intentional effort and practical strategies that allow both partners to nurture their connection while also preserving their individuality. By focusing on specific approaches, you can cultivate a sense of healthy independence while still being deeply connected to your partner.

Establishing Personal Routines
Developing daily routines that include time for self-care, hobbies, and personal interests is a foundational step in maintaining your sense of self. Whether it's setting aside time each day for activities you enjoy independently, such as reading, exercising, or pursuing a hobby, these personal routines allow you to stay connected to your identity outside the relationship. This practice reinforces your autonomy and ensures that your personal growth continues, even within a committed partnership.

Communicating Needs Effectively
Open and honest communication with your partner about your need for personal space is crucial for a balanced relationship. By discussing your boundaries and agreeing on the importance of time apart, you can prevent misunderstandings and ensure that both partners feel respected and valued. Clear communication helps set expectations and creates a shared understanding that personal time is not a threat to the relationship but rather a vital component of its strength.

Planning Time Apart
Intentionally planning time apart can normalize the practice and prevent feelings of neglect or abandonment. This might include scheduling solo activities, spending time with friends separately, or pursuing individual interests that allow you to grow as an individual. By making time apart a regular part of your routine, you reinforce the idea that independence and togetherness are not mutually exclusive but rather complementary aspects of a healthy

relationship.

Encouraging Mutual Independence

Supporting your partner's need for personal space is just as important as advocating for your own. Encouraging each other to pursue personal interests and respecting each other's boundaries fosters a balanced and healthy relationship dynamic. This mutual support helps create an environment where both partners can thrive, knowing that their individuality is valued and their relationship is built on mutual respect.

Practicing Self-Reflection

Regular self-reflection is essential in maintaining a healthy balance between togetherness and independence. Taking time to journal, meditate, or simply engage in quiet moments of introspection allows you to stay attuned to your needs and your emotional well-being. Self-reflection provides valuable insights into your relationship dynamics, helping you to identify areas where adjustments might be needed to ensure that both your independence and your connection with your partner are being nurtured.

By implementing these strategies, you can cultivate a relationship that honors both connection and independence. This balanced approach will help you build a healthier, more fulfilling partnership in which you and your partner can thrive as individuals and as a couple.

Chapter 5 Conclusion

We explored the significant impact of growing up in a toxic family on an individual's perception of independence and personal space within relationships. Toxic family dynamics can instill a fear of independence and foster an over-reliance on constant companionship. These patterns, deeply rooted in a need for validation and security, can severely hinder the development of healthy, balanced relationships.

Understanding the necessity of personal space and time apart is crucial for maintaining both individual well-being and relationship health. Personal space allows for self-reflection, growth, and the pursuit of personal interests, all of which contribute to a more fulfilling and resilient partnership. Time apart fosters independence and prevents the suffocation that can result from constant togetherness, ensuring that each partner retains their sense of self.

We have also discussed practical strategies for achieving healthy independence within relationships. Prioritizing self-care, setting personal goals, and maintaining individual interests are essential steps in cultivating a balanced dynamic. Effective communication, mutual respect, and practicing non-attachment further enhance the ability to thrive both as individuals and as a couple.

By integrating these strategies into daily life, individuals can overcome the fear of independence and the need for constant validation. This empowers them to build stronger, more balanced relationships where personal space and togetherness coexist harmoniously. Achieving healthy independence not only benefits the individual but also strengthens the foundation of the relationship, fostering an environment of mutual respect, growth, and genuine connection.

6. Boundaries: The Foundation of Healthy Relationships

Growing up in a toxic family environment often distorts our understanding of boundaries, leaving us uncertain about how to create healthy, fulfilling relationships. For many of us, boundaries were either violated, blurred, or ignored altogether, leading to confusion about where our personal space begins and ends. In such environments, we may have learned to prioritize others' needs over our own, leaving little room for emotional and mental well-being. Setting healthy boundaries is crucial for reclaiming that space, allowing us to maintain our sense of self while fostering deeper, more balanced connections with others. Boundaries are not just about limiting others; they are about defining what we need to thrive emotionally and mentally.

Healthy relationships require both physical and emotional personal space, enabling individuals to maintain their own identity while remaining connected to their partner. Building on the concept of personal space from the previous chapter, this chapter focuses on how setting and maintaining clear boundaries helps protect that space. Boundaries allow you to assert your needs, avoid emotional enmeshment, and foster respectful, mutually supportive relationships. They ensure that both partners can exist as individuals within the relationship without feeling smothered or enmeshed, providing a structure that fosters emotional safety and mutual respect.

The Influence of Toxic Family Dynamics on Boundaries

For individuals raised in toxic family environments, boundaries were likely neither modeled nor respected. In toxic families, the emotional, physical, and mental needs of children are often dismissed or overridden by the demands and dysfunctions of the family. Personal space and individual needs are either unrecognized or seen as threats to family unity. As a result, children raised in these environments grow up with a skewed understanding of personal limits, making it difficult to establish and maintain boundaries in adult relationships.

In a toxic family, asserting a need for personal space, autonomy, or emotional distance may have been met with anger, guilt, or rejection. This teaches individuals to ignore their own needs and instead prioritize keeping the peace or avoiding conflict. These early experiences can lead to an inability to say "no," the development of people-pleasing behaviors, or a pattern of accepting unhealthy relationship dynamics in adulthood.

The Goal Should Be to Support, Not to Please

One of the most significant mindset shifts for individuals who struggle with boundary-setting is understanding that the goal in a relationship should never be to please your partner but to offer genuine support. The distinction between supporting and pleasing is crucial: support is rooted in empathy, mutual respect, and emotional stability while pleasing is often driven by fear, insecurity, or the desire to control another's emotional state. When the focus is on pleasing, you may find yourself constantly bending to meet your partner's expectations, resulting in emotional exhaustion and resentment when those expectations become impossible to meet.

The need to please often stems from a fear of conflict or rejection, something deeply ingrained in those who grew up in toxic family environments. However, the pursuit of pleasing someone is unsustainable. You cannot control another person's happiness, and making their contentment your sole focus will leave you feeling frustrated and powerless. More importantly, it allows the other person's mood or emotional state to dictate your well-being, which creates an unhealthy dynamic in any relationship.

Offering genuine support, on the other hand, is about providing care, empathy, and understanding while maintaining your own sense of self and boundaries. Supporting your partner doesn't mean sacrificing your needs, identity, or personal space to keep them satisfied. When the goal is to support rather than please, you approach the relationship from a place of mutual respect, where both partners can grow and thrive independently while still maintaining a meaningful connection.

Setting boundaries is essential in this shift from pleasing to supporting. Boundaries protect you from the emotional toll of trying to meet every demand or soothe every mood swing. They allow you to remain empathetic and supportive without losing yourself in the process. For example, if your partner is having a difficult time emotionally, having clear boundaries allows you to offer support without feeling responsible for fixing their emotional state. Boundaries create space for both partners to process their feelings and maintain their emotional health without relying on each other for constant validation or reassurance.

Recognizing and Addressing Boundary Issues

Recognizing boundary issues in relationships is the first step toward change. If you consistently overextend yourself to please your partner, feel responsible for their emotional state, or sacrifice your own needs to keep the peace, your boundaries likely need adjustment. Boundary issues often manifest as feelings of resentment, burnout, or emotional exhaustion because you aren't giving yourself the space and care you need to thrive.

To begin addressing these issues, it's important to reflect on where your boundaries have been crossed or where you have allowed others to overstep. Pay attention to your emotional responses in these moments—feeling drained, frustrated, or overwhelmed are clear indicators that your boundaries need reinforcement. Once you recognize these patterns, you can begin to establish clear limits that protect your well-being while still allowing for emotional intimacy in the relationship.

Communicating Boundaries Effectively

Setting boundaries requires clear and assertive communication. It's not enough to recognize your needs and limits internally; you must also communicate them to your partner in a direct but respectful way. When expressing your boundaries, using "I" statements can help avoid sounding accusatory or placing blame. For example, instead of saying, "You always make me feel overwhelmed," you could say, "I need some time to myself to recharge when I'm feeling overwhelmed."

Boundaries should be communicated calmly and assertively, without fear of how the other person will react. This can be challenging, especially if you are used to prioritizing others' emotions over your own, but it is an essential part of building healthier dynamics in your relationship. It's also important to remember that setting boundaries is not about creating distance or rejecting your partner; it's about protecting your personal space and well-being so that you can remain present and engaged in the relationship.

Respecting Your Partner's Boundaries

Just as important as setting your own boundaries is the ability to respect the boundaries of others. Healthy relationships are built on mutual respect, and part of that respect involves honoring your partner's needs and limits. Encourage open communication about boundaries, and be willing to listen and adjust when your partner expresses their own. Respecting each other's boundaries fosters trust, emotional safety, and deeper intimacy, as both partners feel valued and supported.

For example, if your partner needs time alone to decompress after a stressful day, respecting their boundary by giving them space shows that you value their well-being. Similarly, if your partner expresses discomfort with a particular behavior or topic of conversation, adjusting your actions to honor their boundary strengthens the trust and respect in the relationship.

Enforcing Boundaries with Consistency
Once boundaries have been established, they must be enforced with consistency. Boundaries are not a one-time conversation but an ongoing process that requires reinforcement over time. If your boundaries are crossed, it's important to address the issue promptly and assertively. Repeatedly allowing your boundaries to be overstepped can lead to feelings of frustration and resentment, undermining the health of the relationship.

Enforcing boundaries may involve reminding your partner of your limits or taking steps to protect your emotional well-being when necessary. For instance, if you need time alone to recharge but your partner continues to seek your attention during that time, you might need to reinforce your boundary by calmly reiterating your need for space. Consistency in enforcing boundaries sends a clear message that your needs are valid and deserving of respect.

Chapter 6 Conclusion

Setting and maintaining healthy boundaries is a crucial aspect of creating relationships that are balanced, respectful, and fulfilling.

Boundaries provide the framework that allows both partners to maintain their individuality while fostering emotional intimacy. They protect your personal space and well-being, ensuring that you can offer care and support without becoming emotionally overwhelmed or overextended.

For those who grew up in toxic family environments, learning to set boundaries can be challenging but deeply transformative. Toxic family dynamics often involve blurred lines between individuals, where personal space and autonomy are not respected. By learning to establish clear boundaries, you begin to reclaim your own emotional space, breaking free from patterns of enmeshment and people-pleasing. Shifting the focus from pleasing your partner to loving them unconditionally allows you to free yourself from the emotional burden of trying to control their happiness or avoid conflict. This shift fosters a healthier, more authentic connection where each partner is responsible for their own emotional well-being.

Boundaries also help in healing the deep scars left by toxic family relationships. Growing up in a dysfunctional family often distorts one's ability to form healthy relationships as adults. Without boundaries, individuals can struggle with blurred limits, finding it difficult to separate their needs from those of others. Healthy boundaries allow you to break free from these patterns and redefine your relationships in a way that honors both your individuality and your emotional well-being. They give you the tools to protect yourself from the emotional confusion and manipulation that often emerge from early family trauma.

In relationships, we often rely on automatic defense mechanisms that were developed in childhood to protect us from emotional pain. Without boundaries, these mechanisms—whether it's shutting down, withdrawing, or becoming overly aggressive—become the default response to conflict or discomfort. Setting boundaries allows you to recognize when these defenses are triggered, giving you the emotional space to respond intentionally rather than reactively. By creating healthy boundaries, you can step out of these old, automatic patterns and approach your relationships with greater awareness and emotional control.

Boundaries also play a key role in the process of ego death within relationships. Often, our ego wants to control or dominate situations, leading to power struggles or the constant need for validation. Boundaries help establish a balance between maintaining a sense of self while also embracing vulnerability. They allow you to let go of ego-driven behaviors and approach your partner with empathy, trust, and openness. With boundaries, you can differentiate between what is yours to hold onto and what needs to be released for the sake of emotional connection.

Understanding the dynamics of dependency and codependency also relies on the ability to set and maintain healthy boundaries. When boundaries are unclear, you may find yourself overly reliant on your partner, sacrificing your own needs to maintain harmony. This can lead to emotional exhaustion and resentment. Boundaries prevent you from falling into the trap of codependency by allowing each partner to take responsibility for their own emotional needs and well-being. They provide the structure needed to support healthy interdependence, where both partners are free to grow without relying on one another to feel complete.

Lastly, boundaries are essential for maintaining personal space in intimate relationships. Personal space is not just about physical distance but also about creating emotional and mental room to process feelings, recharge, and maintain your sense of self. Boundaries help carve out this necessary space, ensuring that neither partner becomes overwhelmed by the other's needs. In this way, boundaries foster both individuality and connection, allowing for a healthier balance between closeness and independence.

Boundaries are the foundation upon which all healthy relationship dynamics are built. Whether it's healing from toxic family patterns, overcoming defense mechanisms, releasing ego-driven behaviors, or maintaining healthy independence, boundaries are key to creating relationships that are respectful, balanced, and deeply fulfilling. By setting clear limits, communicating your needs effectively, and honoring your own personal space, you foster connections that nurture both your well-being and the well-being of those around you.

Conclusion: Don't Lose Yourself in Relationships

As we close *Healing Toxic Relationships*, take a moment to reflect on the powerful journey you've undertaken. Healing from the pain of toxic family dynamics isn't just about understanding the past—it's about reclaiming your future, embracing vulnerability, and building meaningful, fulfilling relationships without sacrificing your sense of self. The road to healthier connections begins by addressing the wounds of the past, understanding the ways you've learned to protect yourself, and ultimately cultivating relationships that are both deep and sustainable.

Healing the Deep Scars of Toxic Family Relationships

We began this journey by exploring the deep and lasting impact of toxic family environments. The emotional scars from manipulation, neglect, and abuse shape how we view trust, intimacy, and connection. In toxic families, affection is often conditional and intertwined with fear or control, distorting how we relate to others as adults.

Acknowledging these deep wounds is the first step toward healing. Recognizing how your family's dysfunction shaped your relationships allows you to break free from the unhealthy patterns of the past. Healing involves reclaiming your worth, understanding that you are deserving of meaningful relationships, and releasing the damaging beliefs instilled by early experiences.

Transcending Automatic Defense Mechanisms in Relationships
The survival strategies we learned as children in toxic families—
whether through fight, flight, freeze, or fawn—served a purpose
at the time but now block the deep connections you seek in adult
relationships. These automatic defense mechanisms, designed to
shield you from pain, often prevent true intimacy. Whether it's
emotional withdrawal, confrontation, or people-pleasing, these
patterns sabotage your connections.

But now, you have the power to transcend those defense
mechanisms. By recognizing when they're triggered and
consciously choosing to respond from a place of emotional
awareness, you open the door to more meaningful, authentic
relationships. You can learn to let your guard down, trust, and
connect with others in ways that foster mutual respect and
closeness rather than fear and distance.

Embracing Ego Death in Relationships
Embracing ego death—letting go of the need for control,
validation, or power—opens the door to genuine connection. In
toxic environments, the ego develops as a defense mechanism,
pushing you to seek external validation or control over others
to protect yourself. But this mindset leads to fear, mistrust, and
emotional distance.

Ego death is about releasing those fears. It's about allowing
connection to unfold naturally, without manipulation or control.
It's about being your authentic self in your relationships and
allowing others to do the same. By letting go of ego-driven
behaviors, you create space for vulnerability, trust, and mutual
respect—the true building blocks of a healthy, lasting connection.

Breaking Free from Dependency and Codependency
Growing up in a toxic family can foster patterns of dependency
or codependency, where connection becomes entangled with
emotional enmeshment. These dynamics can lead to imbalanced

relationships, where one person feels responsible for the other's happiness or sacrifices their own needs to keep the connection intact.

Breaking free from these patterns is essential to building healthy, balanced relationships. You can still support and receive support, but in a way that honors your individuality. Healthy relationships thrive on interdependence, where both individuals maintain their sense of self while contributing to the strength of the connection. By freeing yourself from unhealthy dependency, you create space for mutual support and fulfillment without losing yourself in the process.

The Importance of Personal Space in Relationships
One of the key lessons from this journey is the need for personal space within intimate relationships. For those who grew up in toxic environments where autonomy wasn't respected, the concept of personal space can feel foreign or even threatening. Yet, healthy relationships thrive on a balance between closeness and independence.

By carving out personal space, you maintain your individuality while still nurturing your connection with others. This space allows you to grow, reflect, and recharge, ultimately strengthening the bond. Trusting that time apart can enhance your relationships is key to creating a sustainable and resilient connection.

Boundaries: The Foundation of Healthy Relationships
Perhaps the most transformative lesson in healing from toxic relationships is the importance of boundaries. Boundaries are what protect your emotional well-being and personal space. In toxic family systems, boundaries are often disregarded, leaving you vulnerable to emotional enmeshment or manipulation.

Learning to set and maintain boundaries is essential to any fulfilling relationship. Boundaries allow you to connect deeply while still honoring your own needs. They create a framework for mutual respect and emotional safety. Boundaries protect you from overextending yourself and ensure that your relationships are built on trust, understanding, and respect for each individual's autonomy.

Setting boundaries can be challenging, especially if they weren't modeled in your early years. However, it is one of the most powerful tools for creating a relationship where you can connect deeply without losing yourself. Boundaries create the emotional space necessary for both individuals to thrive.

Don't Lose Yourself in Relationships

At the heart of *Healing Toxic Relationships* is this truth: you don't have to lose your sense of self in relationships. Healthy connections aren't about sacrificing who you are or neglecting your own needs for the sake of someone else. It's about creating balance, where you can maintain your identity while fostering a strong, supportive bond with others.

Maintaining healthy relationships starts with honoring your own needs, setting boundaries, and staying true to yourself. When you prioritize your well-being, you're able to show up fully in your relationships without compromising who you are. True connection thrives when both individuals remain whole, contributing to the relationship while respecting each other's independence.

As you move forward, remember that healing is a journey. It requires patience, self-compassion, and practice. Every step you take brings you closer to the healthy, fulfilling relationships you deserve. The insights and strategies you've learned in this book are tools to help guide you on this path.

Your Future is Waiting for You

Healing and growth are lifelong processes. This book has given you the foundation to begin creating the relationships you've always wanted, but the journey continues from here. Every boundary you set, every moment you choose authenticity over fear, and every step you take to honor your own needs brings you closer to the future you deserve.

Don't wait for the perfect moment to apply these principles—start today. Begin by reflecting on the patterns you've uncovered and commit to making small changes, one day at a time. Whether it's setting a boundary, managing a defense mechanism, or allowing yourself the space to grow, every action you take will bring you closer to the life and relationships you desire.

Surround yourself with people who support your growth. Seek out spaces that nurture your healing. This journey is yours to own, but it doesn't have to be taken alone. The encouragement of others will guide you as you continue to build the healthy, fulfilling future you are capable of creating.
Remember, you have the power to create relationships where you can connect deeply without losing yourself. The future is yours to shape—one that is filled with possibility, hope, and endless potential for connection.

Now is the time to act. Embrace your worth, honor your boundaries, and foster relationships that support your true self.

The wonderful and life-changing relationships you deserve are waiting for you.

—*Steven Todd Bryant*

*Excerpt from The Toxic
Family Solution*

The following is an excerpt from Steven Todd Bryant's best-selling book, *The Toxic Family Solution*, available on Amazon.

Journal Part I: Abandonment

Sometimes I wake up screaming. Screaming in a dream is called a *night terror*, a symptom of post-traumatic stress. Trauma is an emotional disturbance caused by a life-threatening or traumatizing event that causes physical or emotional harm. People who have experienced traumatic events, including abuse or domestic violence in toxic families, can experience night terrors. No matter how many years I spend in therapy, I can't seem to make the nightmares stop. I had another one just last week. I've been screaming in my dreams since I was a kid. Perhaps I need to start at the beginning.

When I was eight years old, my father woke me early one Saturday morning. He was about to show me how harmful a toxic family can be.

"Get up. We need to leave right now," he barked at me like a junkyard dog.

I don't remember showering or eating breakfast. Before I knew it, we were in our Volkswagen bus, a cargo van with no back seats. I sat on a World War II footlocker my dad had set up as a makeshift seat for me. The lack of seatbelts in the van seems unthinkable now. I always thought it was strange that my dad had bought a family car with only two seats, one for him and one for my mom. In my young mind, I believed it was a sign he didn't want me around. Later, I would learn I was right.

Mom sat in the front passenger seat. I asked her, "Where are we going?"

"You'll see," she said quietly.

A few minutes later, my dad came to the VW carrying Ruby, the family cat. Ruby was a large black Siamese who followed me like my shadow. I loved her so much. Often, we would cuddle in the sun on our side porch. Ruby mostly lived inside, but we let her out occasionally. My dad handed her to me, and I could tell she was frightened, or maybe I was projecting my own fear.

"Why is Ruby coming with us?" I asked because we had never taken Ruby anywhere in the car. Nobody responded. My mom and dad sat silently as my dad started up the VW. We didn't have a cat carrier, so I held her tightly in my arms and close to my heart. I was her seatbelt.

Dad drove us about a mile from our home in Seattle along the south end of Lake Washington. The sun was beginning to rise just as we passed the local tavern. After turning up a road, we entered a wooded area. Suddenly, Dad stopped the car and ordered me to open the door.

"Let Ruby out of the car. Do it now. Do it quickly so you don't get caught."

"What?" I asked.

With angry black eyes, he yelled, "Do it!"

My dad's tone made it clear that he meant business and

questioning him today would have more severe consequences than usual. Living in my toxic family taught me how to read people. I didn't always know how I felt, but I could always sense the negative feelings in others.

I gently lowered Ruby's body to the ground, placing her on the gravel alongside the road. Tears filled my eyes.

"Don't you dare cry, mister," my father hissed. "Only girls and fags cry."

Under my breath, I said, "This is so screwed up!" I fought hard to stuff my emotions as usual.

"What did you say?" he growled.

"N-nothing," I stuttered in fear.

Dad turned forward, cranked the steering wheel hard, made a quick U-turn, and peeled out of the gravel, kicking up dust all over Ruby's face and body. I looked back and saw Ruby sitting on the side of the road, looking at me as if asking, "Why?"

As we drove away, I looked at both of my parents. Dad looked relieved, but Mom had a dazed look in her eyes.

Once we returned home, Dad went into the basement and began to cut wood with his large table saw he purchased on sale at Sears years earlier. He spent hours cutting wood in the basement but never created anything. I think his destruction of wood was his form of meditation. The dust and noise of the saw filled the house. I felt safe when he was in the basement because I knew where he was, and I could breathe freely for just a minute or two. Mom was doing dishes and staring out the window.

"Mom, why did we leave Ruby in the woods?"

As she gently wiped my cheek where the tears had been, she said quietly, as if in a trance, "Ruby was pregnant."

Anger drowned out my sadness. I ran upstairs and slammed the door to my room. Mom ran behind me and whispered through the door, "Don't ever let your dad see your anger. Not ever."

In my room, I decided to hate my father from then on. Living with my family was nothing but a disappointment. I had to get out of there. I felt hopeless when I realized I was only eight and had ten more years to live in this hell-like prison. Soon after my dad forced me to abandon Ruby and her babies in the woods, I experienced my first night terror and started screaming in my dreams.

A few months later, we were on a day trip to my aunt and uncle's home in Olympia, Washington. My dad was in a bad mood, as usual. Dad got mad because of something my uncle had said and stormed out of their house. We quickly followed behind him, scrambling to get our day bags, coats, and Tupperware containers filled with the food we had brought but hadn't eaten.

Once in the car, my dad wasn't done. He turned his anger on my mom when she started having trouble reading the map. Dad yelled at Mom, ridiculing her for being "stupid" and unable to read "the damn map." Their fight escalated when Mom made a disrespectful comment to defend herself. Dad flipped out and started screaming at her. He slammed on the brakes and pulled the VW into a large hotel parking lot along the roadside.

"What the hell?" I said under my breath.

Like darts, my dad's angry black eyes stared back at me through the rearview mirror. I always tried to be the perfect son, but trying to be perfect never got me out of trouble. The familiar fear and terror I lived with every day possessed my whole being.

"What did you say?" he shouted.

"Nothing. I didn't say anything." I thought to myself, "Don't ever let him know what you are thinking. Don't ever let him know what you are feeling. Don't ever let him see your anger. Not ever."

"Get out of the car right now," he shouted.

"What? I didn't do anything wrong."

"Out of the car now," he demanded.

I knew he was serious, so I got out, and before I knew what was happening, they drove away.

Suddenly, I was standing alone in a parking lot one hundred miles from home. My parents had just abandoned me. In shock, I sat down on the curb. There was nobody to help me. I thought of how my father had told me a thousand times not to talk to strangers or discuss family problems with outsiders and to "always watch out for fags and perverts."

I remembered the story my dad told me about how his dad was a drunk, and his parents abandoned him and placed him in an orphanage at age four. Dad always said they left him there because they didn't love him. As a child, I wondered why my father turned out to be just like his own dad, a drunk who abandoned his kids. I began to wonder if this was also my destiny.

Dad's practice of leaving family members on the side of the road had become a kind of family tradition. A year earlier, Dad got angry and left Mom and me on the side of the road in Bellevue, Washington. I was scared, but Mom took it in stride and said, "We are going to be OK. We just need to start walking home."

I saw her strength while we walked. She began sharing Bible verses she had memorized about how our suffering would make us more like Jesus. She said being left by Dad on the side of the road was a test of our faith, and Jesus would use it to make us stronger. I remember thinking to myself, "Uh, I don't think this is what Jesus had in mind."

This time was different because Mom wasn't there to help, and I couldn't think of any Bible verses. I sat on the curb and stared at my Timex wristwatch my dad had given me for my birthday. Seconds seemed like hours. Many frightening thoughts went through my eight-year-old mind. Hating my dad made the situation seem more bearable. I said to myself, "I'll never let them hurt me again."

When my parents finally returned over an hour later, they didn't speak or apologize. Dad looked angry, and Mom stared straight ahead with a trance-like stare. I knew my relationship with them would never be the same. On the ride home, I began to count how many times my parents had broken my heart. I ran out of fingers and started counting my toes. I remember thinking to myself, "So it's not just family pets who get left alone on the side of the road."

Although I didn't know it at the time, I would live in an abusive and domestically violent home for eighteen years. Nobody was ever physically injured, but much violence occurred. Nobody ever intervened. Nobody ever rescued me. The emotional, psychological, and spiritual damage was fierce and long-lasting.

<u>**The Harmful Nature of Your Toxic Family**</u>
Abuse Is Never Your Fault

Your toxic family caused you to suffer, but it's not your fault. No matter how they treated you, it says nothing about who you are, your value as a person, or your true self. Your unhealthy family's behavior says everything about your family and nothing about you.

No matter how unhealthy your family is, you can overcome whatever happened to you! As soon as you accept the reality of the pain you have suffered, you will begin to feel a sense of freedom. Healing starts with facing the pain, trauma, and neglect you experienced from family members who were supposed to love, protect, and nurture you.

I was shocked when I learned all of the harmful effects of living in a toxic family. Almost every personal and relational problem I have ever experienced can be attributed to the abuse and domestic violence I suffered. As a child, I assumed all families were similar to mine and was unaware my family was domestically violent and abusive. I thought abuse was only sexual and domestic violence was only physical. But I was wrong.

There are seven types of domestic violence and abuse:
1. Emotional
2. Financial
3. Physical
4. Psychological
5. Sexual
6. Spiritual
7. Verbal

If you are being abused or live in a domestically violent home, you need to take immediate action to get help when it is safe to do so. Even if your abuser tells you, "You made me do this to you," abuse is never your fault. No matter what mistakes you might have made, abuse is never your fault. No matter what your family tells you, if you are in danger or are in an unhealthy and unsafe situation, you must take care of yourself and get to a safe place as soon as possible.

How to Get Urgent Help

Abuse and domestic violence are very serious matters and should be addressed immediately. Get help now!

911
- If you are in immediate danger and are the victim of a serious crime, such as domestic violence, abuse, or sexual assault, get to a safe place and dial 911.
- 911 will dispatch emergency medical services, fire, and

police.
- Available 24/7/365

988

- If you are experiencing a crisis, dial 988 for the Suicide & Crisis Lifeline or go to 988lifeline.org.
- You don't have to be suicidal to use 988. Anyone who is in crisis can reach out for help.
- 988 will provide suicide prevention and crisis counseling as well as information about available local resources.
- Available 24/7/365

National Domestic Violence Hotline

thehotline.org

Call, text, or chat 24/7/365

The National Domestic Violence Hotline is a free 24-hour confidential service for victims, survivors, and those affected by domestic violence, intimate partner violence, and relationship abuse.

LGBTQ+ Help

Trevor Project: Crisis Counseling & Suicide Prevention

thetrevorproject.org

Call, text, or chat 24/7/365

Trevor Project is a free twenty-four-hour confidential service for LGBTQ+ crisis intervention & suicide prevention.

Identifying a Toxic Family

What is a toxic family? A toxic family is a dysfunctional family that does not respect the uniqueness of each family member, as evidenced by a lack of respect for personal boundaries. They blame, control, criticize, dismiss, punish, and threaten the people they are supposed to love. Their disrespect often escalates to abuse and domestic violence. Toxic family members enforce harmful rules and force family members to lie, keep secrets, and wear false masks instead of expressing their authentic selves. They judge your thoughts, deny your feelings, and destroy your dreams of a happy life. Substance abuse is also a common problem in toxic families, often manifested in excessive drinking and overeating.

No family member is immune from the damage caused by a toxic family. Rather than loving and caring for you, your family harmed and wounded you. Instead of preparing you for life, they damaged you by preventing you from achieving your maximum potential. They created an environment that robbed you of fully expressing your thoughts, feelings, and true identity.

Characteristics of a Healthy Family
No family is perfect, and every family has some measure of dysfunction. To understand the extent of the damage your family caused you, let's first examine the characteristics of a healthy family. In a healthy family, everyone is loved, protected, nurtured, supported, and cared for, allowing them to express themselves in a safe and healthy manner. Social-emotional development is rooted in love, trust, and the freedom to express your authentic self safely.

Healthy families have the following attributes:
- Authentic self-expression is valued and nurtured, and individuality is encouraged.
- There is clear communication.
- There are consistent rules and rule enforcement.
- Emotional intelligence is practiced and taught.
- Emotional expression is valued and encouraged.
- There are healthy boundaries.
- Healthy conflict management and resolution are practiced.
- Honesty, trust, and mutual respect are modeled, taught, and valued.
- Mistakes are forgiven, and perfection is not expected or required.
- There is no abuse or domestic violence of any kind.
- There is no alcoholism or drug addiction.
- Food is not used as a coping mechanism.
- Outside relationships are encouraged.

- Parents lead by example.
- Problem-solving is accomplished through respectful communication.
- The physical, emotional, and spiritual health of each family member is nurtured.
- Physical punishment is non-abusive.
- There is respect for privacy and personal space.
- Survival skills to live a healthy life are modeled and taught.
- Teaching and training take place in a safe and supportive environment.
- Family members who are struggling with sexual orientation or gender identity issues are loved, guided, and helped with compassion and without homophobia or transphobia.
- There is unconditional love.

Through their words and actions, a healthy family conveys the following messages:
- You are OK, just as you are.
- You are enough.
- It's OK not to be perfect.
- You can overcome mistakes.
- You are accepted despite your weaknesses.
- You have the potential to overcome obstacles and achieve your dreams.
- You belong here.
- There's nothing wrong with you being you.

All of this is possible because a healthy family has unconditional love and trust as its foundation. Healthy family members stand on the shoulders of their healthy families to achieve their hopes, dreams, and aspirations. Healthy families do not shame or punish family members for being different or expressing their authentic selves. In a healthy family, being who you are is never wrong or a mistake. Nobody is perfect. Perfection is impossible. Healthy families accept the authentic uniqueness of family members and nurture them without trying to alter or change their essential nature.

Characteristics of an Unhealthy Family

The following are typical characteristics of unhealthy families:

- There is abuse and domestic violence (emotional, financial, physical, psychological, sexual, spiritual, verbal).
- There is alcoholism or drug addiction.
- Authentic self-expression is judged, viewed negatively, and discouraged ("What's wrong with you?").
- Communication is unclear, one-way, and closed (top-down communication, the parent gives orders, lack of dialogue).
- Emotional expression is not valued and encouraged; primary emotions are sadness, happiness, fear, and anger.
- Emotional intelligence is not encouraged.
- Food is used as a drug or coping mechanism.
- Honesty, trust, and mutual respect are not modeled, taught, and valued.
- Inconsistent rules and rule enforcement.
- Love is conditional.
- Mistakes are not forgiven, and perfection is expected and required.
- Outside relationships are discouraged.
- Parents do not lead by example.
- Problem-solving or problem-resolution skills are lacking.
- The physical, emotional, and spiritual health of each family member is not nurtured.
- Physical punishment is abusive and violent.
- Respect for privacy and personal space is lacking.
- Sexual orientation or gender identity must be heterosexual and gender normative (homophobia, transphobia, heterosexism).
- Survival skills to live a healthy life are not modeled or taught.
- Teaching and training do not take place. (Parent assumes child already knows how to do everything.)
- There are unhealthy boundaries.
- There is unhealthy conflict management and resolution.

Having an unhealthy family discourages the development of who you are, forcing you to guard your heart, question your intuition, and abandon your dreams. Essentially, they ask you to betray and abandon your true self. Conditional love, nonacceptance, and unhealthy boundaries characterize relationships in toxic families.

Toxic families fail to teach you that you are perfectly OK just as you are, negatively affecting your identity, self-esteem, and self-worth. Toxic families punish you for making mistakes and discourage you from expressing your true nature. To survive, you must lie about yourself and others, follow their rules, and suppress your intellectual, emotional, and self-expression.

Even if your family told you they loved you a thousand times and you can remember loving moments you shared with your toxic family, the number of times they hurt you tells the whole story. Displays of love and affection combined with mistreatment and abuse are damaging, confusing, and crazy-making. Despite the sincerity of their love, their good intentions do not justify the harm they caused you. Maya Angelou said, "When someone shows you who they are, believe them the first time." The first time your toxic family harmed you, they showed you who they were. Believe them!

Wounds Caused by Toxic Families

When you realize how much harm your toxic family has caused you, it can be overwhelming. Although each family is different, and toxicity levels vary, the following potential wounds may occur in toxic families:
- Abandonment or fear of abandonment
- Abuse and domestic violence
- Addiction, alcoholism, drug abuse
- Anxiety and stress
- Parentification, where the child is put into a parental role (where a child is made to be a confidant, sounding board, or caretaker or assume parental duties such as cooking

all the meals or being responsible for things a parent would normally do)
- Cognitive distortions or thinking errors such as all-or-nothing thinking, catastrophizing, or personalization
- Codependency (an unhealthy dependence on another person)
- Eating disorders (undereating, overeating, anorexia, bulimia, obesity, unconscious eating)
- Failed external relationships, poor or no relationships outside of the family; a high level of alertness in maintaining external relationships, which is emotionally exhausting
- False sense of reality caused by keeping family secrets and being forced to lie about who you are and how you are feeling
- Fear of being punished just for being yourself
- Feelings of inadequacy
- Fragile sense of self
- Gaslighting (manipulating another person by causing them to question their interpretation of reality)
- Hypersensitivity to invalidation and a constant need for validation
- Humor as a veiled threat or at the expense of others
- Insecurity
- Insomnia
- Isolating
- Job instability
- Lack of authentic identity formation and development
- Lack of emotional intelligence (feelings are limited to sad, happy, afraid, and angry)
- Lack of self-awareness (tendency to blame the outside world for your problems)
- Lack of self-care (self-neglect)
- Lack of self-esteem and self-worth; not valuing yourself, not loving yourself, hating or loathing yourself; lacking self-confidence, self-trust, feeling unlovable or unworthy of love
- Inability to be your authentic self because it feels unsafe (lying to yourself and others)
- Nagging feelings of guilt (you are always in trouble), shame (something is wrong with you), self-blame (what

goes wrong is always your fault)
- Obsessive-compulsive behaviors (avoidance, arranging, checking, counting, isolation, obsessive thoughts)
- Overly self-conscious
- Overthinking and overanalyzing
- Perfectionism (inner self-criticism and the need to be perfect, which mimics your parents' criticism of you)
- Privacy disrespected or ignored
- Prone to hopelessness (belief there is no hope of improving your situation), helplessness (belief there is no action you can take to improve your situation), and depression (low mood with sadness and decreased interest in life activities)
- Prone to repeat dysfunctional relationship patterns learned in the unhealthy family setting in relationships external to the family
- Prone to substance abuse and self-medication to cope with the pain of past traumatic and negative experiences (alcohol, drugs, food, sex)
- Prone to anxiety, fear, stress, and worry
- Rigid, dogmatic, judgmental, and unaccepting approach to self, others, life, religion
- Self-harm
- Sexual orientation and gender identity issues (homophobia, transphobia, heterosexism)
- Shame, a form of self-hatred
- "Should" and "should not" statements
- Suicidal ideation
- Tendency to isolate (avoiding social situations due to feelings of anxiety, depression, shame, or guilt) to avoid further pain (it's easier to be alone or limit relationships)
- Trust issues
- Unhealthy boundaries (either between family members or with outsiders, the words "no" and "stop" mean nothing)
- Use of religion or Bible verses to shame, manipulate, control, or justify abuse and mistreatment
- Control or restriction of access to money
- Symptoms of post-traumatic stress (PTSD):
  - Avoidance, flashbacks, persistent upsetting nightmares and night terrors, recurring

unwanted negative thoughts, and intense emotional reactions to the present moment reminding you of your trauma

My family was highly toxic, and I experienced almost all the above adverse effects. Your personal experience will be different. Regardless of how many or how few of these wounds you experienced, the principles and strategies found in this book will help you move forward toward healing.

Damage Caused by Secrets

Toxic families are full of secrets. People keep all kinds of secrets to survive their unhealthy families. Family members keep secrets for various reasons, but the most common reasons are to avoid pain, humiliation, or punishment. Your family may have kept secrets from each other as well as from people outside the family. Additionally, there may be secrets known only to a few family members or even one member, such as extramarital affairs, financial difficulties, gambling or drug addictions, or issues related to sexual identity and gender non-conformity.

My father regularly warned me never to tell anyone outside of the family about the abuse and domestic violence taking place within our family. For years, I kept secrets to survive in my toxic family, which caused me tremendous fear, guilt, shame, pain, and suffering. I can tell you from personal experience the consequences of keeping secrets for years can be devastating. When you keep a secret, you are basically lying to others about some aspect of who you are. Keeping a secret can be frightening and shameful if you live in a family where they punish liars or are negative, condemning, and judgmental.

Keeping secrets, whether your own or those of your loved ones, can have long-term adverse effects. When you share your secrets with safe, supportive, and empathetic people, they begin to lose their power over you, helping you overcome loneliness, fear, and shame.

The damaging effects of keeping family secrets can include the following:

- Alcohol and drug abuse
- Anxiety
- Backaches
- Digestive problems
- Guilt
- Headaches
- Insecurity
- Isolation
- Lack of well-being
- Low self-esteem
- Obesity
- Self-doubt
- Shame
- Trust issues
- Resentment
- Stress

The first time you share your secrets may be frightening, but you will experience great freedom and relief when you become honest about every aspect of yourself. To reclaim your life, you must find someone with whom you can safely share your secrets. While living in a toxic home, sharing your secrets with your family may not be safe, but I encourage you to find a trusted person outside the family to help you carry your burden as soon as possible. Until you are ready to share your secrets with others, you can write about them in a journal.

Gaslighting

Gaslighting is a form of abuse toxic family members use to control and manipulate their loved ones. Gaslighting occurs when the parent or family member tries to cause the victim to question their sanity, perception of reality, or memories of what happened. The term originated from a 1944 film called *Gaslight*, where a husband tried to convince his wife she imagined things to drive her insane and control her behavior. Gaslighters will create a false narrative to shift the blame for what happened from themselves onto someone or something else. In some cases, gaslighters attempt to convince their victims that what they remember never happened or the abuse they experienced was not as severe as they recall.

The following are examples of gaslighting statements:
- "Can't you take a joke?"
- "Don't be so dramatic."
- "I'm sorry you think that's what happened."
- "I never did/said that."
- "It didn't happen like that."
- "It didn't really hurt."
- "That's not what happened."
- "You're crazy."
- "You're just imagining things."
- "You're overreacting."
- "You're making a big deal over nothing."
- "You're remembering it wrong."
- "You're too sensitive."
- "You're totally misinterpreting what is happening."

Gaslighting is prevalent in toxic families. Every time I tried to raise concerns with my parents about problems within the family, gaslighting was their go-to response. Gaslighting causes the victim to doubt themselves and question their interpretation of reality and makes them feel defective and deficient in their ability to judge and interpret what is happening around them. Gaslighting can cause anxiety and depression, suppress the development of the authentic self, and contribute to psychological trauma. If you suspect a family member is gaslighting you, you can always ask a friend or therapist for a second opinion. If someone refuses to stop gaslighting you after you confront them, you must either walk away from the relationship or keep them at a safe distance.

Roles That Hinder Self-Expression

Family members in dysfunctional homes learn to play roles

they choose or are assigned. Your toxic family prevented you from being yourself, forcing you to wear false masks and play dysfunctional roles to survive. Playing a role and hiding who you are to survive in a toxic family prevented you from developing and expressing your true identity and authentic self. You and your significant relationships outside your family will suffer if you are unaware of these destructive roles and don't act to become your authentic self in all current relationships.

The following are examples of roles family members play in a toxic family:

- Clown
- Confidant
- Enabler
- Golden child
- Scapegoat
- Substance abuser

Clown

Clowns use humor to lighten the family's negative and dysfunctional mood when family life becomes too intense. Clowns believe they can prevent abuse or violence by keeping the family laughing and distracted. The clown will always be on high alert and ready at any moment to elevate the family's mood. Clowns constantly look for changes in the family's emotional state and behavior and thus lose connection with their own emotional condition. Clowns develop a reverse emotional intelligence, where they become highly sensitive and attuned to other people's emotions but not their own. Throughout their lives, clowns will likely be anxious, on alert, and hypersensitive to changes in mood and behavior in all relationships. The clown seeks to help the family at the expense of their own emotional development.

Confidant

Confidants are children who unhealthy parents entrust with their secrets. A parent may use their child as a sounding board, best friend, informal therapist, or a source of advice and support. This role forces the child to provide emotional support, advise the parent, and become the parent's emotional caregiver. Because the child lacks the emotional maturity needed to handle adult issues, they are forced to take on the role of the adult in the relationship, which is called *parentification*. This role reversal damages the child's long-term emotional well-being and is a subtle form of child abuse. Any child who becomes a confidant or feels they need to protect their parent from harm will suffer emotional damage. Confidants learn to ignore their own feelings and neglect their own needs. As adults, they may develop long-term problems such as anxiety, depression, substance abuse, or eating disorders.

Enabler

The enabler helps dysfunctional family members perpetuate and continue harmful and unhealthy behaviors. They may even adopt the same addictive and destructive behaviors to avoid conflict with addicted family members. For example, a wife of an alcoholic may become a heavy drinker to enable and please her spouse. Often in denial, the enabler will overlook the destructive and harmful behavior of the unhealthy family member as well as the harm they are doing to the family. Despite offering a nurturing aspect to the family, enablers can inhibit the ability of the family to resolve problems, heal, or seek help. Enablers frequently repeat this role in relationships outside the family and are often attracted to relationships where they can help or fix others.

Golden Child

The golden child is the family's favorite, the chosen one, the child who can do no wrong. Families treat the golden child as special and gifted. The family celebrates the golden child for their achievements, usually at school or in the community, and overlooks their weaknesses and faults. The golden child feels intense pressure to keep the family together and avoids making mistakes for the good of the family. Even though perfection is unattainable, the golden child often struggles with perfectionism.

Everyone has faults, and no one is perfect. Maintaining a healthy relationship requires accepting the weaknesses and failings of yourself and others.

Scapegoat

In dysfunctional families, scapegoats are the opposite of the golden child. The family blames the scapegoat for all their troubles and bad luck, believing this person is the source of all family problems. The scapegoat serves to distract attention from the real problem, which is the unhealthy family itself. A scapegoat may be the only member of the family who rebels or speaks out, because they believe they have nothing to lose.

Substance Abuser

In many cases, the family's substance abuser is also the head of the family. The substance abuser may also be a child or spouse who adopts addictive behaviors to cope with and soothe the pain of the dysfunctional family. Substance abuse can include alcohol, drugs, food, or any substance used to relieve pain, soothe, and self-medicate. Substance abuse and obesity in dysfunctional families are often multi-generational. Addictions persist from generation to generation despite causing severe health consequences and sometimes death. Those who grew up with a substance abuser may also exhibit similar behaviors, even if they are not addicted themselves. A spouse or child of an alcoholic may also experience symptoms like addiction, including anxiety, mood swings, and depression. If you or a family member is a substance abuser, get help.

Narcissists, Psychopaths & Sociopaths

The following are dangerous roles found in some unhealthy families:

- Narcissist
- Psychopath
- Sociopath

Narcissist

Narcissists have an unhealthy and exaggerated sense of self-importance and believe they deserve special privileges and treatment because they are more intelligent and gifted than everyone else. Narcissists need others to admire them. They dominate discussions, have relationship difficulties, and manipulate people and circumstances. Narcissists do not consider how their actions impact others, lack empathy, and are inconsiderate of the feelings of others. Deep down, the narcissist is highly sensitive to criticism and has feelings of shame, insecurity, and vulnerability, which may be unconscious. Those who live with narcissists over an extended period may experience low self-esteem, question their self-worth, and experience anxiety, depression, and post-traumatic stress.

Setting boundaries is essential when you are in a relationship with a narcissist. A boundary statement may be as simple as, "It's not OK for you to talk to me that way," or, "It's not OK for you to treat me that way." Narcissists may be frustrated by the boundaries you put in place, causing them to erupt in anger. Whenever a narcissist fails to respect your limits, you must decide whether to remain in the relationship or cut ties and walk away.

Psychopath/Sociopath (Antisocial Personality Disorder)
People with antisocial personality disorders (APSD) are also known as psychopaths and sociopaths. Because they are pathologically prone to domestically violent behavior without remorse or guilt, they are the most harmful members of a toxic family. While the chances of having someone with APSD in your family are low, you must be aware of their dangerous behavior.

Characteristics of those with antisocial personality disorders may include the following:
- Few long-term relationships
- Impulsive behavior and failure to meet job and family responsibilities
- Lack of concern about the safety of self or others
- Lack of remorse, guilt, or empathy

- Unable to control feelings of anger

If you believe you are in a relationship with someone with an antisocial personality disorder, seek help from a professional as soon as possible.

Chapter One Summary
The first step to surviving your toxic family & reclaiming your life after toxic parents is to identify the ways in which your toxic family harmed you. In this chapter, we explored how abuse is never your fault, how to get urgent help, and how to identify a toxic family. We discussed the wounds caused by toxic families, damage caused by secrets, gaslighting, roles that hinder self-expression, and narcissists, psychopaths, and sociopaths.